MW00466807

Praise for *BRAIN ON!*

"We often underestimate the strength of the miraculous human brain. Deb Smolensky in this book dives deep into the prefrontal cortex and reintroduces us with vigor and joy to what is possible when we use our heads with intention."

DANIEL H. PINK, #1 *New York Times* bestselling author of *Drive, The Power of Regret,* and *A Whole New Mind*

"Deb understands both the challenges of working in today's world and the opportunities to make it better for both individuals and organizations. *Brain On!* is a great resource to elicit the intrapersonal skills critical to bringing more compassion, energy, well-being, and gratitude into the workplace and workday."

CLAUDE SILVER,
Chief Heart Officer at VaynerX, LLC

"Organizations would serve their leadership and employees well by learning how to apply Deb's mental fitness exercises. *Brain On!* is a playbook to help change work from the inside out."

SCOTT SHUTE, former Head of Mindfulness and Compassion Programs at LinkedIn and author of *The Full Body Yes*

"Deb is doing important work to make organizations of all types work better. We all accept that business performance is a function of human performance—but we don't always invest in the mental health, aptitude, and skills of our people. Deb is working to change that. Her approach, to understand and strengthen the brain at work, is a critical input to better the health of our workforce and our businesses."

ERIC LANGSHUR, Co-Founder and Managing Partner at Abundant Venture Partners

BRAIN ON!

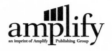

www.amplifypublishinggroup.com

Brain On!: Mental Fitness Strategies for Sharpening
Focus, Boosting Energy, and Winning the Workday

Author photo courtesy of Karla Livney Photography

For more information, please contact:
Amplify, an imprint of Amplify Publishing Group
620 Herndon Parkway, Suite 320
Herndon, VA 20170
info@amplifypublishing.com

Library of Congress Control Number: 2023901374
CPSIA Code: PRV0223A
ISBN-13: 978-1-63755-664-1
Printed in the United States on recycled paper.

Infinite love and gratitude to my incredible husband, David, and daughters, Alyssa and Ashley, for their unconditional love, always believing in me, and cheering me on when I'm at my best (Brain On!) and supporting me and lifting me up when I'm not.

&

To my father, my sister Julie, and Aunt Margie for always encouraging me to follow my dreams.

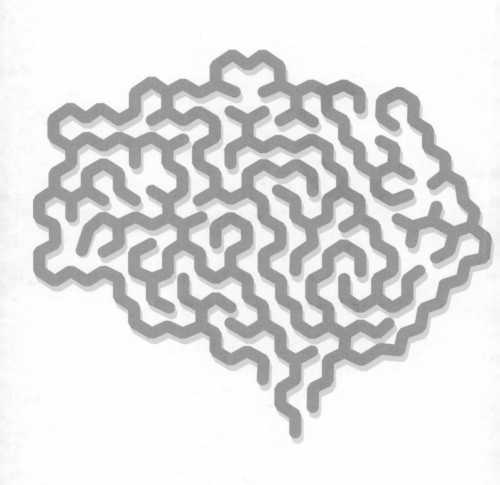

BRAIN ON!

Mental Fitness Strategies for Sharpening Focus, Boosting Energy, and Winning the Workday

DEB SMOLENSKY

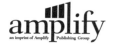
amplify
an imprint of Amplify Publishing Group

CONTENTS

Foreword   1

Game On! Let's Get Started   5

PART ONE Why Your Brain Needs Mental Fitness 13

CHAPTER 1 Your Brain, Version 1.0   15

CHAPTER 2 Your Daily Obstacle Course   27

CHAPTER 3 Brain Energy Management 101   45

CHAPTER 4 Focus Your Energy on Your Strengths 57

PART TWO Brain On! Individual Daily Playbook   77

CHAPTER 5 The New Strengths-Based
Work Goals   79

CHAPTER 6 Six Strategies for an Energizer Day   97

CHAPTER 7 Brain On! Mental Fitness Exercises   111

CHAPTER 8 On-Demand Brain Boosters   129

PART THREE Brain On! Organizational Playbook   141

CHAPTER 9 The Inner Game of Being
a Brain On! Leader   147

CHAPTER 10 HR as the Brain On! Owner   163

CHAPTER 11 Becoming a Brain On!
Regenerative Culture   187

EPILOGUE It's Go Time! Start Winning
the Workday   201

REFERENCES   204

WITH GRATITUDE   207

RESOURCES   211

FOREWORD

It's been over six decades since Peter Drucker coined the term "knowledge worker" to describe the growing part of the workforce that "thinks for a living." Now nearly a billion people around the world are knowledge workers and are the driving force in economic innovation and development.

It has been over two decades since I began teaching my Executive Mind courses, based on Drucker's insight that you can't manage others unless you manage yourself first—starting with your own mind. Systematically learning to manage wayward attention, shift survival reactions, subvert innate human mindlessness, and transform difficult emotions into productive energy is still a woefully rare education for the executive.

Moreover, knowledge workers are also "social workers" since they must work together in diverse teams, cultivate effective relationships, and work in settings where flat and distributed organizations demand a far higher need for skillful communication.

All this is happening as we reexamine important but charged issues of racial justice, sexism, authority, and power while adapting to a warming and unpredictable climate. We find ourselves needing to be effective in situations of tremendous complexity and emotional volatility.

How have we helped workers adapt to these changes? What innovations have we developed to support this fundamental shift from physical work to mental, emotional, and social work? For starters, we created "action offices" (i.e., cubicles) that took away the barriers that foster focus and concentration. We encouraged workers to multitask like the computers on their desks, leading to a depleted mental reserve. We created "always-on" technologies that never let people rest and recharge. Is it no wonder that people are burned out, refusing to go back to the office, or quitting their jobs in droves? Who wants to live like this?

We have failed miserably to take care of the essential foundation human beings who "think (and feel and socialize) for a living" actually need: *their brain.*

Until now.

With profound insight and deep pragmatism, Deb Smolensky has created an accessible, practical, and perennially relevant work. She helps leaders wake up to the reality that has been staring us in the face for more than half a century. Knowledge workers (not to mention all human beings) thrive in environments that support growth, exploration, and development. They shrivel in spaces of fear and threat. Deb's particular genius is to translate these insights into the nitty-gritty of managing in the workday world.

Deb takes on topics that normally get stuck with labels of "woo-woo," "touchy-feely," or the quietly condescending "soft skills," and patiently walks readers through why these are essential for organizations to thrive.

Like an all-knowing aunt, drawing on her decades of experience working with the daily realities of human resource management, Deb spells out in usable language how to implement these tools in your organization. What is their relevance to recruiting, compensation, performance review, and talent retention? What are the questions to ask to open a mind to possibility, learning, and growth? What are the phrases to say to smooth over a difficult situation? Deb gets granular.

Deb decodes something that I've observed over the years. Mediocre managers focus their efforts on their team completing tasks, while extraordinary ones build quality relationships that unleash human energy. The power that is created by safety and trust, humor and kindness, and compassion and supportive challenge is unstoppable. Average is so average because we mindlessly do the wrong things, but where do you ever learn to cultivate transformative individual and organizational energy?

This is a book written by an insider for insiders. It is a practical manual for implementing practices that will jumpstart your organization's morale and performance. At the same time, it's a manual of secrets for individuals who want to adopt strategies that will help them not just survive a chaotic modern workplace but thrive in it with their mental health intact.

Most importantly, as you read through these pages, you will notice the steady drumbeat of what is a revolutionary manifesto for "human resources" in a changing world.

Jeremy Hunter, PhD

Founding Director of the Executive Mind Leadership Institute and Professor of Practice at the Peter F. Drucker Graduate School of Management, Claremont Graduate University

GAME ON!
LET'S GET STARTED

I've spent most of my career focused on mental well-being and human performance in the workplace. I've learned that well-being isn't just about your physical or financial status. The core of well-being is nurturing a strong, healthy, resilient mindset. *I believe the only way to thrive at work is to prioritize mental well-being above anything else.* This is a radically new way of thinking about your workday—taking the steps to ensure your mental well-being is intact before tackling any of your goals for the day and interacting with your colleagues and team.

I've worked with hundreds of major organizations designing strategies and programs for thousands of employees. This experience has given me a whole new perspective on what's wrong with how most of us spend our days in an autopilot, brain-off way. We haven't been taught how to protect and regulate our brain's energy so we can be more productive and happier at work. And it's not just my perspective—there's real science that shows you can train your brain to become more focused, energized, and joyful at work. When you achieve this, you will discover that your relationships become stronger, and you have the energy to sustain growth in your skills and reach your goals. This is where true happiness exists at work and in life.

The brain has always fascinated me, and I'm in total awe of how it works. I'm a neuroscience and psychology junkie and a lifelong learner. The most powerful thing I've learned over the years is that this mysterious, complex gray matter in our heads can be improved and upgraded through mental fitness training that builds up your brain's muscles.

Of course, your brain doesn't really have muscles like your body, but that's how I like to imagine helping my brain become wiser and more resilient. Your brain's muscles become "stronger" as you learn to stay Brain On! and develop healthier and more productive responses to everyday tasks. This muscle analogy is my way of translating neuroscience, psychology, and preventive health into everyday terms and ideas that we can use to develop a high-performing brain.

I like to think of myself as the "Cliff Notes Queen" of mental fitness training. Why? Because I have spent decades studying how our brains perform on all levels in a work environment—physically, emotionally, and spiritually. I explored how our brains work, through both formal learning and lots of personal reading and practice. I searched for answers on how to get more enjoyment and meaning out of work, reduce stress, gain more energy, fuel my passions, and build deeper personal connections.

My big ah-ha moment was when I realized our brains are hard-wired to solve for the needs of the caveman era, not the 21st century, high-paced, complex, challenging world we live in. We all were born with a bunch of primal triggers and responses that can completely throw us off track and shut down our wiser brain. We perceive a lot of daily events and interactions as threats, which result in us getting distracted, overwhelmed, and falling into procrastination, avoidance, fear, and a whole host of other unhealthy thoughts and behaviors. These are the negative results of being in the mental mode of "brain off."

Take advantage of this homework I've done for you! I feel it's my mission to share the brain knowledge I've acquired as well as daily exercises and tips I've developed to stay Brain On! myself and for my clients. My deep wish for you is that this book will help you build a stronger, healthier, and more resilient brain for greater happiness at work and in life.

There's one thing that is true for all of us: Our brains can only focus for a limited amount of time before needing a break. To help me focus, I've adopted the Pomodoro Technique of focusing on a task for twenty-five minutes and then taking a five-minute brain break. This productivity hack has worked very well for me. I suggest giving it a try with this book—twenty-five minutes of reading, and then a couple minutes of reflection time. This technique is also built into many of the chapters. Or take five minutes and relax your brain without any stimulation. No checking social media or the weather forecast for the weekend. Look out your window at a tree or find pictures of nature in your office.

I also suggest reading this book in several sessions. Neuroscience studies have revealed that recall is more effective when your brain has time to process the information through rest and recovery periods, such as a nap, a good night's sleep, or even a vacation. That is when your brain takes the short-term bits of information you've learned and transfers them into long-term memory. Who wants to go through all the time and investment of reading and learning, just to forget it all the next day?

I'll illuminate many of the mental fitness insights and techniques like the ones above by sharing stories from my own life. I'm going to be vulnerable and let you in on my experiences and my own mental well-being journey. I hope my stories will help inspire and guide you in how to develop a new relationship with your brain and your-self—a relationship built on deeper understanding and compassion as you seek to become your best self at work and in life.

Your relationship with your brain will never be perfect. But in this book, you'll discover many effective mental fitness techniques, practices, and habits to keep your brain healthy, fit, and working for you, not against you. Ultimately, this will allow you to win your workday.

BRAIN CHECK: You just spent about five or ten minutes reading the previous paragraphs. How many times did your mind jump to thinking about something else? The email waiting for you to answer, the call you need to return, the pressing errand to run, or the bills coming due for payment. No judgment here—it's just a fact of modern life. We are all juggling a million details between work and our personal tasks. Our brains simply can't keep up. They don't have storage and bandwidth for all this nonstop input. So, what happens? We end most of our days feeling emotionally drained, unfulfilled with our work performance, and just plain stressed and burned out.

We've done our best to design *Brain On!* in the most brain-friendly way possible—through readable fonts and use of white space in the design and engaging use of illustrations and color. Still, staying in the moment is difficult. Throughout the book, look for brain check activities like this one. They are a great opportunity to check in with how you are practicing Brain On! in a given moment. Consider these brain checks to be opportunities to "get your reps in" and stay ahead of the workday.

Flip the Script

This book is divided into three parts designed to "flip the script" on how to become mentally resilient at work as an individual and an organization. Parts One and Two are structured to help individuals at work, and Part Three then expands these lessons to anyone in a leadership or HR position. You'll discover that being Brain On! is what transcends any performance goals, team incentives, or bonus plans in creating engagement at work.

Part One starts our journey by discussing why you can change the relationship with your brain, the leading neuroscience and psychological thinking on how the brain works, and why conscious awareness of your brain's on-off state can result in more productive and happier workdays.

Part Two is the Brain On! Individual Daily Playbook, where I outline proven ways to keep your brain focused and moving toward your goals. You'll learn how to create your own mental fitness routine that will train your brain to use effective techniques, practices, and habits to get you through the obstacles you encounter at work.

Part Three is the Brain On! Organizational Playbook designed specifically for leaders, HR teams, and the overall organization to keep employees Brain On! and to create a thriving environment. If you currently don't lead or manage people, work in the HR department, or are responsible for organization-wide programs and communications, you may not want or need to read this section. If you aspire to be such a leader, I suggest keeping this book on hand for when you do become one.

My goal is to help you end each day feeling happier than you were the day before and ready to face the next day with more awareness, optimism, motivation, and resilience. We can never eliminate challenges and obstacles completely. Those are just a given in life. But you can develop an inner response mechanism that allows you to address and express your emotions around work issues in healthier ways. Achieving Brain On! prevents you from feeling like you are always churning and burning at work. You will stop wasting precious energy on meaningless tasks and start using it to succeed at your goals.

Ready to get your brain in the best shape of its life? Let's get those cells moving and the conversation started!

Meet Onyx

Incorporating healthy habits can be a challenge, especially when you can't always see the results of your hard work. When you break a bone, you can feel it heal and see your muscle tone getting stronger as you go through rehabilitation and exercises. But with your mental fitness workouts it will be hard at times to notice that you are becoming stronger and more mentally fit.

When it comes to starting any new healthy routine, such as Brain On!, I like to visualize things, so I've created this character, Onyx, to represent your brain and what it might be thinking as we introduce new ideas.

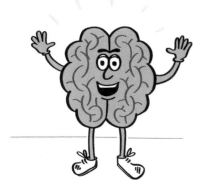

We all tend to be so hard on ourselves and our behaviors, so I hope Onyx will inspire you to view your brain and yourself with greater understanding and more self-compassion.

PART ONE

WHY YOUR BRAIN NEEDS MENTAL FITNESS

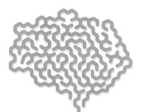

Are you often stressed at work with too much to do? Do you get frustrated with the futility of playing catch-up with your inbox? Can't find time for the bigger, more fulfilling projects because you're running around putting out one fire after another? For most of us, the solution is to power through all our tasks at any cost to ourselves, our team, and our organization. But this way of working leaves us exhausted at 5 p.m. every day, unmotivated to start again the next day, and eventually burned out.

Here's why: your brain gets easily tripped up and turned "off" by all the daily distractions and obstacles that pop up. No matter how "smart" you may be, your brain isn't built to process all the thousands of pieces of information coming at it each day. When your brain feels overwhelmed, it stops its healthy "thinking" mode and defaults to the more primal "emotional" mode. That's when we start making poor behavior choices and unwise decisions that can have lasting and destructive consequences for ourselves, our team members, and others in the organization.

I bet that's something you've never thought of before—how you can help your brain regulate its emotions to avoid falling into negative or unproductive thinking. Some people talk about this training as rewiring your brain. I like to think of it as upgrading your brain to a new version that is much better suited to help you meet your goals at work and the demands of life. I want to help you move beyond reacting with the primal, emotional part of your brain to staying Brain On! and ensure you have the most engaging, productive, and fulfilling day possible. It took me a long time to grasp this concept. Much of my life I didn't understand why I was reacting a certain way at work or in life, and why that led me to feeling anxious, frustrated, or just in a funk. I didn't understand that if I changed the way my brain reacts, my day at work—and my life—would change for the better.

To do so, I realized I needed to develop my mental muscles and strength through mental fitness exercises and workouts. I'm going to share how I became mentally fit, and how you can, too.

CHAPTER 1
YOUR BRAIN, VERSION 1.0

"Why do I get so off track?"

Our brains are the most powerful yet archaic "technology" that we possess. The brain doesn't come with a "user manual." Few of us were taught about mental well-being in school. We learned plenty about our physical body and anatomy in health and gym classes but little about how our brain functions or how we can keep it in tip-top shape from an emotional standpoint.

And here's the real kicker: Our brains haven't had an "upgrade" since the beginning of time. There hasn't been a release of Brain Version 2.0 or 28.0 or 999.0. Our brains still function primarily as they did for our ancestors who walked the earth thousands of years ago.

Like our cave dwelling ancestors, your brain is designed mainly to keep you *safe*, not to keep you *happy*. Yes, your brain pretty much wakes up every morning thinking its job is to be your protector and act like your bodyguard fending off big (and little) threats. It's not built to be your best friend, be calm and compassionate with you, give you good advice on dealing with relationships, or how to accomplish your daily goals at work. Once we understand that the brain's function is primarily as a protector, it's easy to understand why we aren't happier, calmer, and more present throughout the day. Ever wonder why you were so mad at someone, or afraid to make a mistake, or anxious about public speaking? It's your brain operating in its primal or brain-off mode. It's doing what it was originally designed to do. Keeping you safe and alert. Warning you of dangers and threats. Unfortunately, the brain was not wired to keep us in the present moment and joyfully humming along, but instead it is always scanning the horizon for problems. (If only our brains could live by the motto "Don't go looking for trouble where none exists.")

Your brain's primary organizing system is to sort every input or stimulus into two buckets: threat or reward. That means our brain's default is to consider everything as either 1) potentially causing harm or even death, or 2) being an innocent and safe interaction for us. We all operate with this basic sorting system, and it governs a great deal of our behavior. Neuroscientist Evian Gordon refers to this as the "minimize danger, maximize reward" response.[1] When you encounter something unexpected like a shadow in the corner of your eye, or a new and unknown co-worker moving into the office next door, the limbic part of your brain (the more primitive and emotional part that we share with most animals) is aroused. While that sounds like an efficient way for a brain to handle all the "data" it's receiving, it does not serve us well in today's complex and nuanced world.

Your brain spends most of its day operating as a prediction machine, taking very seriously its role and responsibility in looking ahead to keep you safe. It is basically hardwired to do one thing: be on the alert for any new, strange, uncertain, or threatening situations. It does so through pattern recognition, memory recall, and past experiences. For example, when you drop your phone, you probably react quickly in a fearful way because you think your phone is now damaged. Your response is automatic and subconscious, and you create hundreds of these predictions—and fear-based reactions—every day. Your brain reacts at hyperspeed to a stimulus and makes an instant assumption, and often an incorrect and negative one.

For example, about five years ago I was taking my daily walk through the forest preserve by my home, and I saw a coyote ahead on the path. I instantly froze, and then quickly made a beeline for home. My brain did its job—kept me safe from danger. However, still to this day, when I see a large animal off in the distance, I automatically freeze and feel a slight pang of fear in my chest for a second. Until I realize most times that it's a large dog and I couldn't see the owner behind a tree. No coyote at all, but my brain's initial instinct is "threat ahead." Our brains and bodies go through that predictive (and mostly inaccurate) analysis hundreds of times a day. These moments of real or perceived threat release the hormone cortisol in our body, which is part of our built-in alarm system response. Too much cortisol in the body, however, can lead to anxiety, depression, and loss of energy and concentration. Not a great way to live your life at work or at home.

> BRAIN CHECK: When in the last few days did your brain make a "threat" prediction that turned out to be something minor? Did you think you lost your keys, went into panic mode, but then found them in your coat pocket or bottom of your bag? Did you think you sent an email, but it was still in your draft folder, and you were worried that your response was too late? Did you see your boss calling you at the end of the day, and start to fear you didn't meet a deadline, only to find out it was just about a simple question? Think about what your initial physical or emotional reactions were to situations like these. Did you feel yourself tense up or your heart speed up? Simply being aware of our brain's natural threat predictions, and slowing down our response to them, can keep us calmer and healthier during the day.

As sophisticated and marvelous as the brain is on many fronts, it hasn't evolved to truly process more than a couple pieces of information at a time, as Daniel Levitin explains in his book *The Organized Mind.²* Our cave-dwelling ancestors only had to deal with a suspicious rustle in the bush a couple of times each day, or maybe an occasional loud noise from a dinosaur, saber-toothed tiger, or grizzly bear. In the fast-paced, information-based world we live in, our brain is overwhelmed at the millions of pieces of information we take in each day and the decisions we need to make. And we are talking millions—Levitin says *our brain takes in over 11 million pieces of information every second unconsciously and only forty bits of information consciously.* No wonder we are all exhausted by 2 p.m. and running for a caffeinated beverage or a handful of cookies to try and boost our energy.

As Levitin emphasizes, we are only consciously aware of about 0.000001 percent of the information in our world. This leads to hundreds of internal, unconscious, emotional reactions, assumptions, biases, attitudes, and judgments all influencing your mood and day. They're also influencing your sense of choice, what you think is possible, how you react to things, and eventually the happiness and other positive results you get during the day. Just knowing this fact alone helps me realize why energy management is critical and our "brain power" is a precious resource (more about this in Chapter 3).

With all this information coming at us, it's extremely difficult for our brains to stay focused and pay attention. Distractions are ever present and keep us off-track more than on-track. There is significant scientific debate about how long we can really concentrate and focus on a task, but most research seems to agree that after ninety minutes, your productivity will start to decline. This basic rest-activity cycle (BRAC) was proposed by Dr. Nathaniel Kleitman, a sleep researcher at the University of Chicago back in the 1930s.[3] Other research since then also supports that fact that people perform best with ninety minutes of work, followed by a twenty-minute rest period. This gives your brain a break and helps maintain its power.

There are dozens of moments in our day when the demands of the modern workplace can trigger our primal and predictive response. Do you cringe when you see a certain phone number come up, thinking it's your client, customer, or patient calling with a problem? Find yourself feeling frustrated when someone sends a document back again for the twelfth time, assuming there are more edits you must make because it's not right yet? Get a text from a co-worker asking for more time to finish the project? All these little "threat" moments during the day can shut our wise brain off, and we start to react emotionally based on past experiences and patterns. Our goal is to be smarter about how we manage our thinking and responses and maintain our mental well-being throughout the day. Key to managing ourselves and our well-being is mental fitness training which you'll learn a lot about in Part Two.

Brain-off Example

My phone rings and I see it's my daughter's school calling. My initial reaction is never one of glee, joy, or calmness. Within a split second, before even saying hello, I've decided (that is, my brain has predicted) that my kid is hurt, sick, or got in trouble, and my body is immediately armed and ready to jump into action. If I pay attention, I can sense my heart rate is up, I hold my breath, my shoulders and muscles tighten, and I've clenched my jaw prepared for the "blow of bad news." Ugh. Only to find out, literally ten seconds into the call, it was nothing.

It was simply that I forgot to send in a form, or they forgot their lunch or homework. Okay, time to take a breath. After a predictive event like this, most of us never take a moment to consciously calm down, relax and process what happened. And we wonder why our necks are stiff, our back hurts, we have a heart attack early in life. Our environments and stimuli are so complex and fast paced, our brains are always in a hyperalert mode. This type of prediction and then assault on our body and mind happens hundreds of times a day. I jump from one perceived crisis to another. The minute I hang up from the school, I check my email and see my boss sent a message asking me to call her when I have a chance. I have a great boss, so you'd think I'd remain calm. No way. Again, my brain predicts there is something wrong, and I'm back in panic mode assaulting my body all over again. The reality is she simply had a question about a report. One wrong prediction or fear-based response after another, and another, and another. All day long. Creating more stress and exhaustion. Good grief!

Luckily, there is a natural feedback loop built into our brain-body connection. We can update our prediction model using these wrong guesses to change our responses in the future. But our brains are ancient technology we are working with, so this updating doesn't happen very quickly and not without mental fitness training and tools. Even now that my girls are in college, if the school calls, I get a knot in my stomach assuming the worst has happened with them.

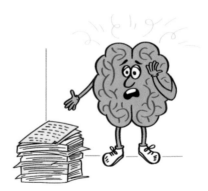

When it turns out to be a noneventful call regarding the tuition bill or fundraising request, I still need to peel myself off the ceiling and calm my heart down, take some deep breaths, and remember what the heck I was working on or where I was at in an important work conversation. Really?!?! We are all works in progress when it comes to keeping ourselves Brain On! and I'm no exception. Progress over perfection continues to be a helpful refrain for me.

As humans in the 21st century, we want and deserve more out of life. We don't want to be at the mercy of every little piece of information or unexpected communication coming at us. We want to feel happy, maintain calm, be productive, and to not be triggered by perceived threats big and small throughout the day. In this book, you'll learn how to work with the brain's innate programming to reshape and rewire it. Think of it as upgrading to a new version of your brain, just as you do with your phone or computer. When you upgrade your brain and strengthen it to be mentally fit, I promise you that this will lead to more resiliency, joy, and energy at work.

The good news is the brain can change. Science proves we can rewire our brains. This concept is called neuroplasticity. I was first introduced to the idea of neuroplasticity in Dr. Jeffrey Schwartz's book *Brain Lock.*[4] The key concept in this book is called self-directed neuroplasticity and is referenced in many of the leading personal development, self-help, productivity, and performance books. Dr. Schwartz gave me hope that I could reprogram and rewire my brain in ways that could help me overcome my obsessive and compulsive habits and irrational thoughts. Other books that were pivotal in helping me get more mentally fit include *Change Your Brain, Change Your Life* by Dr. Daniel Amen[5] and *Hardwiring Happiness* by Rick Hanson.[6]

Take a minute for self-compassion here. No one has taught you how your brain operates, especially at work, how it gets in your way during the day, and takes you off course much of the time. Think back to your health class or gym class at school, and how you had to learn the muscles of the body, what they are for, and how to make them stronger. We're going to do the same thing now with the brain by reviewing its structure, the different parts, and how it functions (in a simple and brain-friendly way!).

The easiest way I know how to explain the brain's structure, for purposes of our mental fitness training, is to use Dr. Dan Siegel's hand model of the brain.[7] He is a world-renowned neuropsychiatrist and uses this model to explain to parents and kids how our brain is built. It's also a great tool to understand how we get angry or frustrated when the emotional brain takes over the thinking brain.

Here's how you can picture your brain's parts:

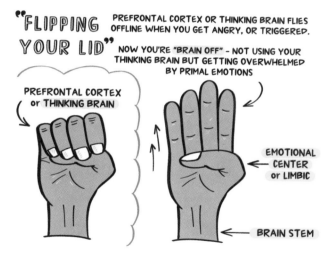

"FLIPPING YOUR LID" PREFRONTAL CORTEX OR THINKING BRAIN FLIES OFFLINE WHEN YOU GET ANGRY, OR TRIGGERED.

NOW YOU'RE "BRAIN OFF" – NOT USING YOUR THINKING BRAIN BUT GETTING OVERWHELMED BY PRIMAL EMOTIONS

PREFRONTAL CORTEX or THINKING BRAIN

EMOTIONAL CENTER or LIMBIC

BRAIN STEM

- Hold one hand up and facing you.
- The wrist is your brain stem.
- The thumb is your emotional center or limbic, and it easily folds and flexes into the hand.
- Wrap your fingers over your thumb, and that is the prefrontal cortex or thinking brain. The prefrontal cortex flies offline when you get mad, angry, or triggered, and now

you've "flipped your lid" and are brain off. This means you are not using your thinking brain but instead are getting overwhelmed by your primal emotions.

Before we can work on mental fitness strategies, we need to understand in more detail the brain's different regions and what they are used for. Think about how you tour a fitness center before joining or starting a new routine to learn how to strengthen certain muscles with certain machines. We're going to go on a tour of your brain in the same way, learning how to strengthen these "muscles" with different mental fitness routines. Stay with me here—this will be a lot easier and more fun than the typical science class!

There are two main regions of your brain for you to know about— the emotional brain and the thinking brain. ***Here's the key thing to remember—these two parts can't both be "on" at the same time.*** Guess which one part is on most of the time? Hint: it's the one that is scanning the world for threats. Our default mode is to the emotional brain and its fight-flight nature. That's what gets us in trouble because our default mode = brain-off mode.

The Brain On! mode is our thinking brain or the prefrontal cortex. This is what keeps us in a rational, wise, and conscious operating mode throughout the day. It's where our best decision-making and problem-solving happens. The prefrontal cortex is extremely important because it manages all those critical skills like comprehension and planning. Neuroleadership expert Dr. David Rock's *Brain at Work*[8] explains that the prefrontal cortex is the biological seat of your conscious interactions with the world. It's the part of your brain central to thinking through things, instead of being on autopilot. He clearly outlines how critical this region is for our happiness and success, as it controls how we:

- Understand (and are open to new ideas)
- Make decisions (compare and choose between two things)
- Recall (information from memory)
- Memorize (take in information and hold on to it)
- Inhibit (keep other nonrelevant thoughts out of our working memory)

Our prefrontal cortex is always competing with the emotional center of our brain and especially the amygdala. This part of the brain elicits our emotional responses. In today's complex world, our amygdala is on hyperalert and responding in that fight-flight-freeze routine. Over and over, all day long. Wearing our energy down until we feel edgy and unhappy.

> BRAIN CHECK: Quick, how are you feeling right now in one word? Happy, sad, angry, tired? Can you even describe your emotion? Most of us automatically respond quickly instead of taking time to assess how we are really feeling. Research shows that less than a third of people can tell you what emotion they're experiencing in any given moment. Psychology once assumed that most human emotions fall within the universal categories of happiness, sadness, anger, surprise, fear, and disgust. But a study from Greater Good Science Center[9] suggests that there are at least twenty-seven distinct categories of emotions. Within those categories, there can be dozens

of distinct, identifiable emotions. Why is it important to be able to identify our emotions? As author and researcher Brené Brown says in her book *Atlas of the Heart,* "When we name an emotion of experience, it doesn't give that emotion or experience more power, it gives US more power."[10] The more we can name emotions, the more we are able to regulate them.

Your amygdala and this abundance of emotional responses doesn't have to be a runaway train, however. Emotions aren't hardwired into your brain at birth. They are constantly being formed throughout the day. Here's the good news: *We can use our brain to manage and create the emotions we want to experience at work.* This is probably one of the most empowering sentences you will read in this book. Having emotional regulation is at the core of being mentally fit. In the following chapters, you'll learn strategies and techniques to keep you in a highly energized state—one where you are open to learning and growth and feel more positive about your future at work.

BRAIN CHECK: Okay, before heading into Chapter 2, you'll want to check in with yourself and make sure you're Brain On! and ready to learn more. Or do you need to take a quick break and give your eyes and brain a little breather from all this information? Take a moment, once again, to notice your energy level. Are you tired, energized, hungry, thirsty? If so, take a quick stretch break. Or even just one minute to reflect on what you've learned and how you can apply that learning in your daily life. This will help give your brain a quick reset and refresh and be ready to learn more.

CHAPTER 2
YOUR DAILY OBSTACLE COURSE

"Geez, why can't I get anything done?"

D
o you wake up most days with an anxious feeling because you're afraid to look at the day's calendar? Does reading those overnight texts and emails give you a stomachache before you even have your morning coffee? Your poor brain hits the ground running each day with all kinds of tasks, conversations, meetings, and emails all waiting to be dealt with. Then it's sideswiped with all kinds of unexpected demands during the day from big things like a last-minute change to a presentation that's due to a client, a sudden issue with an important customer, or a text requiring immediate attention. No wonder we all feel like contestants on the *Survivor* television series,

where we are trying to battle the elements. Most of us don't face physical obstacles at work like needing to hunt for our lunch or fending off a wild animal, but the survival course for all of us in today's work world is just as emotionally challenging and grueling.

Each of us has a different daily obstacle course at work depending on our roles, responsibilities, and skills. We all are required to perform several functions throughout the day, usually in the form of tasks, meetings, and conversations. But here's where things go off the rails: We get sidetracked by all kinds of emotional and psychological obstacles and distractions that take up more time in our day than the actual work itself. Think about that. Dealing with these challenges and distractions can take up more than 50 percent of your day. Imagine how much more productive we could be, and how much more time we could devote to long-term goals that we want to accomplish, if we could just handle these obstacles in a less time-consuming and energy-sucking way. When you are operating in brain-off mode, you are operating on autopilot and going through the motions dictated by your calendar or email inbox. Brain-off mode leaves you feeling less energized and engaged in your work.

As much as we try to intentionally plan out our workflow for the day, we get easily thrown off by two types of obstacles:

Internal obstacles are the thoughts, stories, and feelings that influence the perception of your environment. They influence the choices you have, which then influence the actions you take, ultimately influencing the results you achieve each day. The limbic part of the brain (your survival and protection system) is creating these internal obstacles, which are really the emotional drivers responsible for how well we handle our daily obstacles.

External obstacles are the interactions you have with other people and the environment around you, such as co-workers, clients, and vendors. The quality of these interactions has a big influence on your daily experience and energy level. So do your encounters with environmental obstacles such as bad lighting, a noisy office, ergonomic discomfort, a cluttered desk, or even the lack of tools or resources that you need to get your job done. Any of these external obstacles can take your brain offline and get in the way of you doing your best work each day.

Sample of a brain's typical workday obstacle course:

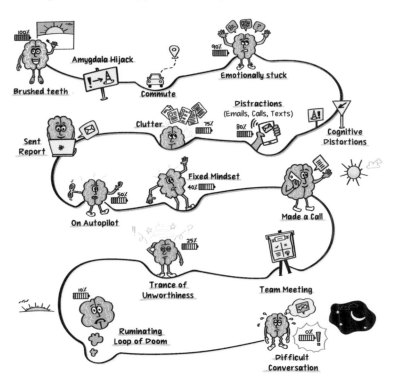

We create most of our own obstacles and problems ourselves because of the internal thoughts, emotions, and stories we are telling ourselves. Mark Twain's quote really opened my eyes to this important concept. He said, "I've had a lot of worries in my life, most of which never happened." I'm going to give you a quick review of some of the common internal and external obstacles to be aware of during your workday. Take a deep breath—it's not that you will experience all of these in a single day or week, but over time, it's likely many of them show up without you noticing.

Internal Obstacles

STUCK IN NEGATIVE EMOTIONS

In her book *Real Happiness at Work*, world-renowned meditation teacher and author Sharon Salzberg describes the five categories of negative emotions that can plague us during the workday: desire, aversion, sleepiness, restlessness, and doubt.[11] Desire itself isn't the problem—it's when we get over-attached to the results. Aversion is a strong reaction based on fear, impatience, and anger. Sleepiness is really the manifestation of switching off or disconnecting, which happens when we're overwhelmed. Restlessness shows up as anxiety or worry, and doubt keeps us stuck and unable to make decisions. Too many negative emotions, or ones that go on for weeks or months, prevent us from finding joy and meaning in work.

AUTOPILOT BEHAVIOR

Research shows up to 90 percent of our daily actions and behaviors are on autopilot. We are like pilots who flip the switch, so the plane flies itself, or we're motoring around like we're in a self-driving car. That is exactly what happens when our thinking brain is off, and our emotional brain is running the show. A great example is you are driving to work or the store, and you arrive in the parking lot and suddenly wonder, "how did I actually drive here safely?" You don't really remember anything about the drive. The brain is built to conserve energy, so it takes shortcuts from thinking consciously. Our brain doesn't want to think about how to perform a task every time we do it, especially for those tasks that become habits or are repetitive patterns. We walk through our entire day, very unaware and unconscious of every reaction and decision we make.

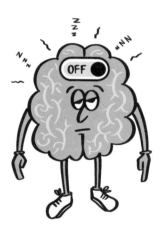

WANDERING MIND

There's a difference between daydreaming and a wandering mind. Daydreaming is a stream of consciousness that can lead to creativity and problem-solving. A wandering mind is when your brain goes off-roading from what you are currently doing and spends too much time scanning for threats or new things to divert your attention away from a focused task or being productive. When your mind wanders, it is often into a bad territory of worry, self-doubt, irritation, or fear. Your brain deserves a break during the day, but the trick is to notice when it goes off-track and meanders into unhealthy and negative fields. Science shows your brain will mind wander close to 50 percent of the time.

RUMINATING ABOUT THE PAST

Ever lie awake at night, replaying over and over an event that happened at work that day? A disagreement with your boss, a snide remark from a team member, or a look of disappointment from a client? When we are feeling under stress, we often tend to rewind our mind and replay the event. It feels as though we are on a never-ending rollercoaster. It's not productive and sucks the joy right out of us. Dr. Amishi Jha, professor of psychology at the University of Miami, and author of *Peak Mind,*[12] calls this the "loop of doom" where we spin the same content over and over in our minds. Have you ever said something in a meeting and then for hours later replayed that conversation in your mind, getting down on yourself by asking, "how could I have said that!" or "why didn't I speak up?" That is ruminating. Your brain can't tell the difference between a real-time event or one replaying in your head. Every time you keep ruminating about that past situation, your brain (and body) responds as if it's occurring in that present moment. You assault yourself over and over when you ruminate.

TRANCE OF UNWORTHINESS

We live in a culture of constant comparison that is provoked by social media images of perfection and constant press focused on billionaires and unicorn start-ups. It's a wonder any of us can muster up enough positive energy to face the day. Tara Brach, author of *Radical Compassion*, calls insecurity the "trance of unworthiness." We all go through periods where we feel we aren't good enough, smart enough, qualified enough, confident enough, pretty enough, tall enough, and the list goes on and on in our head. This kind of thinking stops us from taking chances; following our dreams, passions, and interests; and using our voice for change or to make things better.

These thoughts at times have been huge obstacles in my growth and pursuit of health and happiness. They have held me back from applying for new opportunities, suggesting new ideas, and having the confidence in my own skills to speak up in a meeting when a leader or expert is in the room. I have come to learn that this is normal, my brain is just trying to protect me from what it perceives as a threat. I now know that my fears are not my truth, and these thoughts don't represent what I'm capable of achieving. But this trance of unworthiness can really do a number on your self-confidence and your ability to take risks, learn something new, or pursue what makes you happy.

PARALYSIS OF UNCERTAINTY

This is one of the biggest triggers for our brain. As we've learned, the brain is a predictive machine that seeks quick answers, and it hates the stress of uncertainty. Over time, this ongoing stress affects your ability to focus and remain productive. Let's face it, there are only a few things that we can be certain of in our lives—there are always emails to answer and taxes to pay. In fact, the world we live in today can be described as VUCA— volatile, uncertain, complex, and ambiguous. Think of a time when you couldn't solve a problem, or you couldn't find that answer. You couldn't stop thinking about it, because the brain needs to find answers, close the loop, predict what is a threat to your survival. Your brain faces uncertainty hundreds of times a day.

Uncertainty at work is a constant challenge that stops you in your tracks, leads to procrastination, or has you defending your position on a topic for fear of the unknown outcome. During the day, uncertainty can be part of your decision-making obstacles because you fear what will happen if you make the wrong decision. It can even lead to having a brain-off mode about the future of your job and your health. Uncertainty may have stopped you from changing your investment in your 401(k), or even investing in your future, for fear of the unpredictability of your financial situation tomorrow, or in a month.

WORKPLACE BIASES

You can't really be a human without having biased thoughts. It's impossible to walk through this journey and be 100 percent perfect and making the most inclusive decisions at every moment. That's just not how being human works.

UNCONSCIOUS BIAS. This happens to everyone. It's when your background, personal experiences, and cultural context have an impact on decisions and actions. Unconscious bias happens when we make snap judgments and assessments of people and situations without us realizing. Though sometimes quick decision-making can save time and energy, sometimes knee-jerk reactions lead to bad choices.

DISTANCE BIAS. At work this obstacle surfaces in many ways. Our distance bias is when you are in an office, and you have a question that needs an immediate answer. Your brain automatically looks for someone close by versus someone who is most knowledgeable. Promotions or heading up a project can happen this way too, when someone is tapped on the shoulder who that manager "sees" instead of someone who is equally qualified but not as visible.

EXPEDIENCE BIAS. Your expedience bias is when you are in a hurry, and you go with your gut decision without pausing to gather facts or do more research.

SIMILARITY BIAS. This is when you believe people like yourself are better than others, and this can create group think, where everyone shares the same opinions and beliefs. Solutions then become "one-sided" based on how you all collectively think versus having diversity of thought on your team or for a project.

BRAIN CHECK: Let's bring this to life. Take out a piece of paper and list three to five people you would contact to discuss a problem with or ask for help on a work matter. The people you list cannot be close friends or family. Now, next to each name, put the following information:

GENDER _____

AGE _____

RACE _____

GEOGRAPHIC LOCATION _____

Now just look at the list you've created. How similar is it to you, your background and life? Most of us will come up with a list of people that are like us. Unintentionally, most of your biggest supporters, mentors, or co-worker confidants are probably very similar to you. That is just how unconscious bias works unless we strengthen our mental muscles and train our brain to pause, before automatically knocking on the office next door, or calling someone like us for assistance. Otherwise, we will miss out on getting the best, most applicable, and diverse input and support.

LACK OF CURIOSITY

Our brain is an organ in our body that uses a lot of energy (more about that in the next chapter). To conserve energy, our brains rely on matching patterns to assess situations and make decisions. This can automatically shut down our curiosity, which shuts down our innovative and creative thinking. Lack of curiosity can stunt your career growth by stifling your learning. It can also detract and degrade your relationships with team members and customers. If we don't take time to be curious at work, we often fall prey to not making things better (process improvements), and not making things more efficient or better for us. Our fear brain inserts this obstacle because curiosity and questioning make us think. It uses brain power (energy). You get so busy that you just plow through your task list head down and brain off to get through your day. Asking good questions and flexing your curiosity muscle helps you adapt, create things, improve things, and understand things and people in new and helpful ways.

FIXED INSTEAD OF GROWTH MINDSET

Your mindset matters more than you might imagine. Stanford psychologist and researcher Carol Dweck[13] discovered that having a fixed or growth mindset plays a critical role in determining a person's success. Simply put, a fixed mindset is one that doesn't believe in changing, adapting, or improving skills, while a growth mindset is a belief that skills can be improved over time.

When you have a fixed mindset about a topic, situation or person, or obstacle at work, it can limit your thinking and the choices you make. You might not seem flexible or adaptable to work with because you come off as stuck in your ways. You may come across as ultra-conservative and unwilling to take any risk, which could hold the team back from a project or starting a new initiative. Or people might not see you as a team player because you don't take chances or have that curious mindset when you are in a fixed mindset mode of operation. It's important to notice when you are displaying thoughts and actions based on a fixed mindset because those thoughts can be a big obstacle for you in accomplishing tasks, learning new approaches, and building great working relationships.

WHAT KIND OF MINDSET DO YOU HAVE?

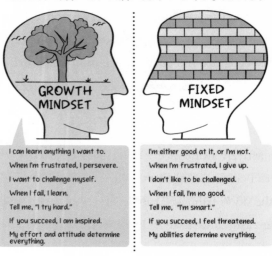

GROWTH MINDSET

I can learn anything I want to.

When I'm frustrated, I persevere.

I want to challenge myself.

When I fail, I learn.

Tell me, "I try hard."

If you succeed, I am inspired.

My effort and attitude determine everything.

FIXED MINDSET

I'm either good at it, or I'm not.

When I'm frustrated, I give up.

I don't like to be challenged.

When I fail, I'm no good.

Tell me, "I'm smart."

If you succeed, I feel threatened.

My abilities determine everything.

COGNITIVE DISTORTION

This is a big one, at least for me. A cognitive distortion is an exaggerated thought pattern without any basis in fact. Unfortunately, these exaggerated thoughts are primarily negative, and very convincing in getting you to believe negative things about yourself and daily life situations. An occasional cognitive distortion is part of being human, but too many of them too often takes a toll on your mental well-being.

Some common cognitive distortions:

- Making everything into a catastrophe.
- Jumping to conclusions.
- Need to always be right.
- Overgeneralization.
- Discounting the positive.

Just by reading this list, you can probably guess the ramifications this type of thinking can have on your projects and work relationships. It leads to undue stress and alarm, negative communication, and inability to recognize the good and see all that you accomplished. For me, I need to be aware of my tendency to have catastrophizing thoughts. Being a type-A perfectionist, I don't always handle issues as calmly or clearly as I'd like. It is one of my more difficult obstacles. I am actively aware of it and working to change my response. Sometimes I catch myself acting like Chicken Little and responding as if the sky is falling. This turns out to be just a small problem that can be easily addressed if I just breathe and be Brain On! again.

BRAIN CHECK: Take a minute to pause, observe nature, or find something that makes you smile or laugh.

External Obstacles

We also have numerous external obstacles that cause our brains to go offline and off-course from what we want to accomplish and how we want to show up in our day. These are just a few of the detrimental ones.

DISTRACTIONS

Anything that is new, a novelty or a change in our environment, attracts and engages our amygdala and our "alarm system" to figure it out. That is one of the reasons why we are so addicted to our phones, to the news, to social media. Our brain has learned that good news sometimes comes in the form of an email, text, or social media (so it triggers our reward system and of course then we want more). Unfortunately, many of these external and tech-driven distractions convey negative information or waste time, which doesn't serve us well in terms of our well-being, productivity, or relationship goals.

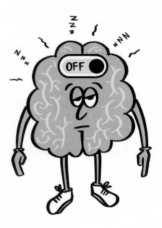

DIFFICULT CONVERSATIONS

Renegotiating a contract. Not seeing eye-to-eye with a co-worker on a decision needing to be made. Providing feedback on a less-than-stellar project. These are all necessary conversations to produce high-quality work and grow a team and a business. It's our emotional perceptions and reactions to them that cause us to categorize them as unpleasant, difficult, and something we'd love to avoid if we could. On top of our own negative experiences, it's our fear of the other person's reaction, of which we have no control, that can derail the ability of our brain to function from a place of calm.

This external obstacle can halt us from using our voice to improve the situation or circumstances at work. It can lead to many sleepless nights trying to figure out how to approach a person so they don't get mad or offended. Or we avoid people or meetings altogether because we just want to avoid any conflict. And unfortunately, what we do not address early seems to fester until it creates a very uncomfortable and stressful working environment for you and everyone around you. Being in default, fear-based mode never ends well. There is rarely a situation when you ignore a difficult conversation and it all fixes itself and everyone is happy again.

BRAIN CHECK: We've covered a lot of ways that our brains go offline during the day. Which of these internal and external obstacles have you experienced today? In the last month? Take two minutes and list as many examples as you can:

Internal obstacles | External obstacles

_____ | _____

_____ | _____

_____ | _____

_____ | _____

_____ | _____

Stay Aware of Your Brain's Response to Obstacles

Your brain's job is to manage these inner and outer obstacles using emotional regulation. We need to train our brain to be aware of when the "threat" or alarm system is going off and make sure the wiser, thinking part of the brain is on for healthier responses. Here's a simple tip to remember: *When you manage the inner obstacles first, this will lead to successful management of the external ones.*

Keep your brain from being hijacked by your amygdala continually throughout the day. This is how you can tell your brain has been hijacked:

- You're exhausted, burned-out, or just have low energy
- You get rattled, frustrated, angry, annoyed easily
- You are worried, anxious, freaked-out and can't focus
- You snap or are abrupt with someone
- You interrupt someone who is speaking
- You regret what you did or said after the dust settles
- You blame, shame or guilt someone (silently or publicly)

When your amygdala hijacks your brain, you experience inner chaos and rigidity, and your emotions start to snowball out of control. Your workday starts going south within seconds because of unhealthy responses.

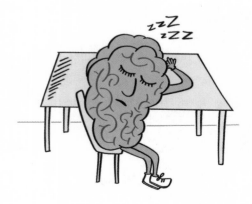

Inner chaos responses	Inner rigidity responses
Blame	Delay
Worry	Depression
Panic	Sadness
Frustration	Apathy
Impatience	Disconnection
Racing thoughts	Giving up
Impulsiveness	Giving in
Anger	Ignoring
Rage	Denying

Again, show yourself and your brain some compassion here. You haven't been trained until now to be aware of your daily obstacle courses and how your amygdala can easily hijack the thinking part of your brain. We all have felt the energy-depleting ramification of poor emotional responses, and it's why we are ready to just collapse on the couch at the end of the day with a fuzzy blanket or cold beverage and binge watch our favorite show to escape it all. Your job is to manage your emotional responses to stay energized throughout the day and enthused about starting the new one. We're going to learn all about energy management in this next chapter.

CHAPTER 3

BRAIN ENERGY MANAGEMENT 101

"Why am I so exhausted?"

I hope you've given your brain a break from all the information it absorbed in the previous chapter. Now take a minute to review the obstacles you outlined in the chapter. The purpose of going through these obstacles is to demonstrate that you are asking your brain to run a marathon every day—and it's not an easy or flat course! There are dozens of "brain-breaking" hurdles, steep hills, muddy pitfalls, and overall rocky ground that require a high degree of awareness to keep moving beyond and forward. It's like you're participating in a Tough Mudder extreme challenge every day. The amount of energy it takes to do that day in and out is enormous.

But your brain is a limited resource when it comes to the level of energy available. Think of it as a huge battery pack that needs to be plugged in and fully charged to perform at its best and last throughout the entire workday. And some days are more energy depleting than others. Your job is to stay aware of and monitor how fast your brain power is draining, and carefully and continuously redirect energy toward those goals and tasks that lead to more productivity, growth, and joy. The strategy is like when your cell phone is losing power and you have less than one bar left. You probably wouldn't waste that remaining power by randomly scrolling through your social feed or streaming a show. Same goes for your brain—managing your brain's energy takes awareness and skill.

Although the average brain only weighs about three pounds, it uses 20 percent of your body's energy. The problem is most of that energy is wasted on negative thinking and fear-based responses. There is much debate about how many thoughts we have in a day, but most scientists agree it's into the thousands. Most of these thoughts are either negative or repetitive from the day before. Stop and consider that for a minute: Most of your brain's energy is spent on responses based on your default mode of survival—ready to fight, flee, or freeze.

No wonder many of us wake up each morning not terribly excited or energized by the prospect of hitting the daily obstacle course again. We haven't been taught that almost 100 percent of our day is driven by our unconscious, autopilot mind. We're unaware of how unaware our brains are working (read that sentence again so you're fully aware!). Our subconscious or brain-off mode is controlling almost everything we do each day.

That's why it's so critical to be aware that your energy gets depleted with negative and unhealthy responses, which then distorts your thinking, and your day turns into one filled with worry, angst, problems, arguments, and burnout. You aren't conscious that your brain has switched over to unconscious mode, and suddenly, you find yourself responding like one of your Neanderthal ancestors. Once your battery pack starts draining, you become less enthused about your work and less engaged in it. You just don't have the fuel to keep on going. But consciously and strategically boosting your brain power during work will keep you Brain On! and more productive and engaged.

> BRAIN CHECK: Based on what you've learned in this section, it's sobering to know that in the last five minutes, you probably only retained 50 percent of what you read. You were distracted or your mind was wandering more than eight times, and you probably didn't even realize it. You may have looked around the room. You may have checked your phone a few times for emails or texts. Got up to stretch or get something to eat or drink. No judgment, it's your subconscious brain overriding your thinking, fully focused brain.

The simplest way to describe being Brain On! is being aware of how your brain is acting and responding. If you don't have brain awareness, you can't manage your workday successfully. It's like trying to drive down the freeway with a dirty or foggy windshield. You just can't see things clearly.

When you are fully energized and Brain On!, you'll experience more positive feelings such as:

- Optimism
- Calm
- Balance
- Peace
- Happiness

- Gratefulness
- Focus
- Playfulness
- Fulfillment
- Inspiration

Who wouldn't want more of that!? The payoff for committing to and regularly doing your mental fitness practices is enormous. It's one of the only ways you can add more joy, productivity, and purpose to your work and life.

> BRAIN CHECK: From the list above, jot down two of those words that you want to experience more of at work and why. These two words will help fuel your motivation for committing to and consistently doing your mental exercises. We all need motivation and goals to achieve success, and this is where your mental well-being success story starts.
>
> 1. _____
>
> 2. _____

I want you to keep showing yourself and your brain some compassion because what we don't know, we can't change. And it's extremely hard to stay aware when your day and energy start to go south. It happens mostly subconsciously and in split seconds. Pat yourself on the back for how far you've come in using your brain in a highly complex way in today's modern work world. And just think how far you'll go once you learn how to strengthen your brain muscles, keep energized, and stay Brain On!

Each of us is a product of our own emotional genetic makeup, environment, and past (often unpleasant) life experiences. Add in the predictive nature of our brain and we can easily find ourselves brain off. For example, even though we are excited for a new opportunity, new client, or even a new co-worker or manager to join the team, our brain goes back to the first day of school or being in a new school. Will they like me? Will I be accepted? Who will I eat lunch with or sit next to at a conference? What if they make me participate in that dreaded ice breaker? And before you know it, you are completely worked up, can't sleep, and go through a million different scenarios in your head just because of old programming and file cards in our brain, and the fact our brain considers these situations as life-threatening when rationally we know they are not.

Our brain's new responsibility is to show up in every moment with awareness. The goal is to check in with yourself regularly throughout the day to make sure you aren't brain off, just going through the motions, jumping from one meeting or task to another on autopilot. When this happens, you can't see the situations or tasks clearly, objectively, or rationally. Working in brain-off mode makes you feel unproductive, stressed, and less joyful about your work.

Brain On! is when you are working consciously and strategically in handling the day's events, using mental fitness techniques, practices, and habits to stay energized and enthused about your work and achieving your goals. That is the endgame of being Brain On! —it's activating a high degree of mental and emotional regulation to keep your energy at its peak and feel true joy and engagement in your work.

At every moment, our thinking, wise brain is either off or on. And based on how our brains are built, which is to keep us safe not happy, our thinking brains are off most of the time, causing feelings of being overwhelmed, exhausted, fearful, angry, in conflict mode, and resulting in poor performance during our workday. Remember—only one mode can be on at a time. If your brain is offline most of the time, running on autopilot and subconscious programs, your decisions, interactions, and performance will also be subpar.

Are you brain off or Brain On!?

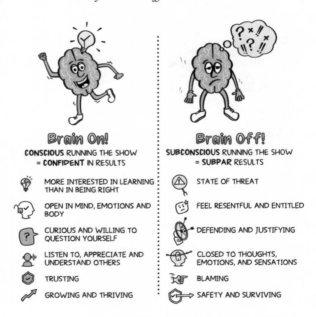

Brain On!
CONSCIOUS RUNNING THE SHOW
= **CONFIDENT** IN RESULTS

- MORE INTERESTED IN LEARNING THAN IN BEING RIGHT
- OPEN IN MIND, EMOTIONS AND BODY
- CURIOUS AND WILLING TO QUESTION YOURSELF
- LISTEN TO, APPRECIATE AND UNDERSTAND OTHERS
- TRUSTING
- GROWING AND THRIVING

Brain Off!
SUBCONSCIOUS RUNNING THE SHOW
= **SUBPAR** RESULTS

- STATE OF THREAT
- FEEL RESENTFUL AND ENTITLED
- DEFENDING AND JUSTIFYING
- CLOSED TO THOUGHTS, EMOTIONS, AND SENSATIONS
- BLAMING
- SAFETY AND SURVIVING

You can use this illustration to check in throughout the day to better understand which state you are currently operating in. When checking in with your brain, ask yourself: Am I using my thinking (conscious) brain or am I using my emotional (unconscious) brain right now? Basically, is my brain off or am I Brain On?

How can you assess how much energy is in your brain's fuel tank to help you stay focused and productive? To do so, I've created four states of "brain energy" that most of us encounter throughout a day, week, a month, or a year.

THE BRAIN ON! ENERGY MATRIX

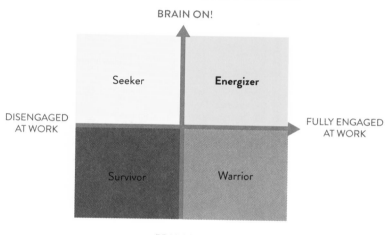

The goal is for your brain to be in Energizer mode as much as possible during the day, and on as many days as possible. The other energy states represent your brain during the moments, days, or weeks when you are veering too off course and losing energy and engagement at work. I'm not talking about the caloric energy your brain needs from food, but rather the energy state of being fully charged instead of depleted. It's the difference in the energy we feel when we are engaged in our work, or just going through the motions.

ENERGIZER

"I accomplished so much today. I'm feeling good and ready to tackle tomorrow!"

This is your target. You have the highest level of mental fitness because you remained Brain On! and don't fall into crisis mode even when faced with challenges throughout the day. By having the highest level of energy and focus, you accomplish more, find more meaning in your day, feel a sense of belonging and connectedness, and can spend more time on goals you want to achieve. This is what gives you more happiness and engagement work.

SEEKER

"Something's off today, and I'm not feeling the spark about work."

Maybe you've been in a position for a while, a project is dragging on and on, or there's been too much grunt work lately. You feel unfulfilled. Because you are mentally fit and aware of your thoughts and feelings in this quadrant, your Brain On! response is to think strategically and not fall into a fight or flight mode. You recognize that you need to take healthy actions and find a way to align work with more passion, joy, and interests.

WARRIOR

"I like my job but am feeling stressed out and burned out."

Did you cruise along on autopilot all week, getting a million things done, but not really feeling much joy? Or practicing good self-care? You might be hyperproductive or even just pushing through to the point of not taking breaks, eating lunch, or other techniques to give your brain battery a rest. You may not be checking in with yourself enough, pumping the brakes to evaluate the quality of your thoughts, feelings, and relationships to ensure the next day (and the next day) is more fulfilling. The question you need to ask yourself if you stay in this state for too long is "will I survive my own success?" And at what price? My health, my relationships? All work and no play make for a very brain-off day that is depleting and unhealthy.

SURVIVOR

"Work was nothing but problems, and I couldn't wait for this day to end!"

You felt like you were constantly being bombarded by people and situations at work that made you angry or frustrated. Everyone and everything seem to irritate you, and you couldn't catch a break. You were doing tasks that weren't meaningful or aligned with your interests. Your thinking brain shut off and was operating almost 100 percent from your limbic system, causing unpleasant and unhealthy emotional responses. You found yourself constantly in flight-or-fight mode, which leaves you anxious, depressed, and unhappy at work. You feel like you are barely surviving, or even suffering, at work. Some call this a clock watcher, and the minutes seemed to just drag on.

BRAIN CHECK: How energized are you today, or this week? Reflect for a couple of minutes on which of the four energy states best describe where you spent most of your day. And if you weren't in Energizer mode, write down specific internal and external obstacles that have prevented you from being in that quadrant.

If you are in Energizer mode – that is great to hear. Reflect on why you are there. Can you think what you have strategically and consciously done to stay focused and engaged at work and how to build those items or habits in each day to ensure it becomes part of your daily routine?

After reflecting on which energy state(s) you found yourself in this week, please be kind to yourself, especially if you fell into the brain-off mode of Survivor or Warrior more times than not. Unlike looking into a mirror or having a doctor's exam to determine our physical fitness, we don't have a way of "seeing" or assessing our mental strength and well-being. But the good news is there are mental fitness exercises and tips to upgrade and improve our brain's strength and resiliency that you'll learn in Part Two. The even better news (in my opinion) is that this isn't something you have to carve out time for, unlike changing clothes, driving to a gym, and doing some crazy exercise routine with complicated equipment. You are already using your brain all the time, just not training it in all the right ways, to build those new mental muscles. It's about your brain working smarter, not harder. It's about regulating your brain, so you won't be depleted at the end of your workday but feeling re-energized and ready to start in that same positive mode tomorrow. Imagine that?!

Let's revisit the statement I made in Chapter 1:

We can use our brain to manage and create the emotions we want to experience at work. I said this may be the most empowering sentence you will read in this book. In this chapter, we've seen why creating an Energizer experience is what you want to aim for each day. The benefit of being in an Energizer state is that your day is devoted more to showcasing your strengths and skills, instead of merely ticking off a to-do list and reacting to fire drills.

CHAPTER 4

FOCUS YOUR ENERGY ON YOUR STRENGTHS

"How can I stay in Energizer mode?"

You've learned why staying in the Energizer Zone is your goal throughout the day. How do you accomplish that in the middle of what feels like a million to-dos and distractions? It starts by identifying the unique strengths you bring to the workplace and using your energy to let those strengths flourish and grow.

No matter what our professions or job titles, we all want the same thing: To be happy, feel like we've accomplished our tasks and made a difference, and enjoy the people who are on our team. Making a difference you feel proud of—whether you're just starting out in your career or are at a senior level—starts by knowing your strengths or "superpowers" and using them to be at your best each day. When you plug into these internal gifts and talents it keeps you more energized, motivated, and engaged at work. If your strengths can't shine at work, it's unlikely you'll be as happy and as interested in your work, and just plodding along will negatively impact your energy levels. Being clear on your strengths and how you want to use them gives you a sense of direction and purpose. Purpose is the foundation of engagement at work. It gives you the intrinsic motivation to keep you focused on what you want to achieve for yourself and your organization. And ultimately it helps keep your brain battery fully charged and raring to go.

For me, I saw the value in identifying and using my strengths long ago. I've taken many formal assessments to help clarify my strengths and understand the context in which to use them. No matter which assessment I have taken, each one reveals that my strengths and passion revolve around creating things that are innovative and inspire people. Innovation and Inspiration are my superpowers, and when I remember to use them (Brain On!) I feel more energized, motivated, and fulfilled. For example, I created this book to inspire you to adopt this innovative approach of mental fitness at work to help you thrive each day. When this project became challenging or overwhelming, my strengths and purpose were what gave me the energy and motivation to push through.

Many of us are given specific performance goals to meet at work, whether it's a sales figure, client retention or acquisition rate, or profitability percentages. Your purpose at work is deeper than that—it's how you see yourself making a true difference in the lives of your clients, team, organization, and of course, yourself.

When you know your purpose at work, it gives you the ability to apply your strengths to those projects and activities that are most fulfilling to you, again helping you achieve the Energizer state.

Engagement Influences Better Well-Being

A Gallup study[14] showed that people who are engaged in their work have entirely different experiences with happiness and stress. Those who were engaged enjoyed significantly higher happiness levels throughout the day. And were happier even on nonworking days. Those who were disengaged had the opposite experience. Their stress levels were substantially higher, and happiness only increased at the end of the workday. Why spend so many hours and days of your life more stressed and less happy? Identifying your purpose and strengths and applying then to your work will positively influence your well-being 24/7.

There are many terrific books and assessment tools on how to find your purpose and identify your strengths. I've compiled a list of some of my favorite resources here: www.debsmolensky.com/resources. Some of you may be familiar with tools such as CliftonStrengths Assessment, which identifies your innate, natural talents so that you can invest in them through practice to make them your strengths. It's a simple formula to remember: Talent x Investment (Practice) = Strengths.

I am a big fan of Tom Rath's book *Life's Greatest Question: Discover How You Contribute to the World.*[15] Rath, who is an expert on human behavior and a senior scientist at Gallup, explains that "our real job is to figure out how to make the greatest contribution through our job." Rath believes that it is up to each of us individually to "figure out how to make purposeful contributions."

There are no "perfect" jobs in life, but Rath believes as I do that "most every one of us can start by maximizing the contributions you are making in your current role." You can't maximize your contributions if your brain is off (and taking you off track), but only when fully energized and Brain On!

A simple example to make this point is to consider a professional team sport. Each person made the team because they have certain strengths, gifts, and talents that collectively can help a team achieve a winning record. However, when an individual player is benched or doesn't get any playing time, that player may not feel very engaged anymore. They are still contributing by supporting their team from the sidelines, but their main purpose and contribution isn't being maximized. Same is true for you. You likely have those days when you must perform those menial tasks. Or you found yourself excluded on a high-profile project or from an important meeting. These are the days you might fall back into Seeker or even Survivor mode.

It is possible to turn the job you have into the job you want at every moment. Through research for his book, Rath discovered that contributions in a workplace could be described in three universal words: Create, Operate, and Relate. Let's use that three-word approach to think about your unique strengths and contributions in the workplace.

> BRAIN CHECK: I want you to spend a few minutes brainstorming three words to describe your strengths, gifts and

talents, contributions, and your unique superpowers. You don't have to find a perfect word, and down the road, you may find a new word that gives more clarity and depth to how you enjoy applying your strengths at work. Here are three quick techniques to help get at your three-word description:

TECHNIQUE #1: HIGHLIGHT REEL

Look at your "highlight reel." Look back into your past and write down experiences you've had at work that you really enjoyed or when you felt you made a difference. Those days when you were really in an Energizer state. Think about what these experiences may have in common. Did you inspire something new? Did you go above and beyond in service to your team or client? Were you the one keeping people's spirits positive during a particularly tough or busy time? Come up with a list of experiences here, and jot down some words that explain the common theme between them:

TECHNIQUE #2: ASK SOMEONE WHO REALLY GETS YOU

Ask a colleague, friend, or family member to help uncover the theme. Choose a handful of people who really know you and have seen you in different situations. These people will have an objective and often surprising view on your strengths, and what you have been admired for throughout your life. For example, my husband had not considered his purpose and strengths until I was writing this book. After talking through his highlight reel, we discovered his purpose is "to have fun." His first instinct, like so many, is that can't be right. "That doesn't seem significant enough. My purpose is to have fun?" After we discussed it, it became obviously fitting since he is always the one in our house making us laugh and offering ideas to have fun together as a family. He creates that same environment at work for his employees where hard work and fun go hand in hand to deliver superior client results. At the end of the day, he is a consultant in what many consider a very stressful industry, which further highlights the importance of using your strengths to create the positive experiences and results you want. By incorporating this strength into his life and business, he strategically aligns to things that bring in joy as much as they do success.

TECHNIQUE #3: IDENTIFY WHAT BRINGS YOU JOY

What do you enjoy doing each day? If you don't have the opportunity to regularly do something you enjoy, the odds of you having high career well-being are lower. And sometimes the things you enjoy doing may not be the job task themselves. I always enjoy catching up with a colleague about a project they are working on or events in their personal life. You may find talking to a friend or family member during your lunch break or to and from home can be the enjoyable part of your day. Even spending those breaks learning something new or reading a good book counts. Whatever you enjoy during your day, whether it's a specific skill directly used at work or something you do on your breaks or outside of the task at hand, all will lead to you identifying your strengths.

Those activities might equate to broader strengths such as building connections, collaborating, creating, being of service, caring for others, learning—all which can be applicable to your work. Tom Rath notes that people with a higher career well-being are more than twice as likely to be thriving in their lives overall. He goes on to explain that "people with high career well-being wake up every morning with something to look forward to doing that day. They also can do things that fit their strengths and interests."

YOUR THREE STRENGTHS

I used several of these techniques and came up with the words Inspire, Create, Innovate. (I was a little influenced by some of my assessment results, as you can tell). These words have become my North Star and main energy source at work and at home, too. Looking back, it is obvious that when I wasn't aligned with my strengths, my health, motivation, relationships, and career all took a hit.

For example, before I knew the importance of doing work that interested me and aligned with my strengths, I struggled in my career path. I graduated college as an accountant and worked for a large private bank handling the budget and forecasting of five major departments. I absolutely loved talking to my clients and helping them, but I didn't find joy in the actual work, and struggled to figure out why I was not happy and engaged. I was in Seeker mode. Looking back, only one of my key strengths and passions was being met – inspiring people. However, there was not enough opportunity for me to be creative or innovate in my job. I left the bank to join a large consulting firm that offered me more opportunities to incorporate these additional strengths.

But this time, in this fast-paced consulting world, I operated in the Warrior state. I hadn't built my mental muscles to realize my sixty-hour work weeks were leading me to a path of significant burnout, bouts of anxiety and depression, and physical pain. I loved the job and the people, so I kept pushing forward until I ran out of gas and fell into Survivor mode where I realized I no longer liked how I was feeling or the work I was doing.

After I left the consulting world, I started my own business. I had young kids who wouldn't eat their vegetables, and at the time sneaking those brightly colored foods in kids' meals was all the rage. So, my sister-in-law and I created a frozen vegetable puree company – Hip Hip Puree! For a long time, I was in Energizer mode, given I was using my strengths, aligned to my purpose, having good success. But, when it came time to expand our business and invest significant capital, I finally checked in with myself. I didn't even realize that deep down I wasn't truly engaged in this work. It seems I was fluttering between Seeker and Warrior, rarely Energizer. I remember this really catching me off guard.

How could I not be in Energizer mode when I'm creating all the time (new products, new client bases, etc.) and inspiring people (moms always writing in saying thank you for Hip Hip Puree!)? After much reflection, I figured it out. Being in Warrior mode most of the time, I just kept pushing through, building the business, but my brain was off. Once I took a timeout and did some self-care and deep reflection, I was Brain On! again (moving into Seeker mode). In that state, I put two and two together: I absolutely hate cooking. I was so excited and motivated about the possibility to create a new, innovative product that helped people, I didn't even realize that what I'd be doing most of the days was cooking puree. That was not energizing to me!

That is how powerful aligning to your strengths and purpose can be. But it can also lead you up the wrong mountain if you don't check in with yourself and build your mental strength.

My two big lessons to you from my experience:

- Be as clear and detailed as possible about what you like, what interests you, what your talents and gifts are, so that you can hone in on and align to those things that best match up.

- Don't wait years, months, or even days before checking in with yourself. Pausing and reflecting throughout the day so you can course-correct can significantly improve your life.

Those were hard lessons for me to learn and took years for me to realize, but the experience also was a catalyst for me to implement the daily check-in and to take charge of constructing my own reality, moment-by-moment, as often as I can.

Be Aware of Emotionally and Socially Sabotaging Your Strengths

Remember the concept of internal and external obstacles (or challenges) I discussed in Chapter 2? We reviewed those obstacles in the context of your day or week at work. Here I want to introduce you to some of the ways we sabotage ourselves both emotionally and socially at work. These saboteurs, or voices in your head, are the negative and repetitive thoughts, feelings, or behaviors that can truly block your ability to use your strengths and maximize your contributions.

EMOTIONAL SABOTAGE

The ongoing scripts and dialogues we play in our mind can disrupt our ability to be Brain On! Maybe you've heard that phrase "the stories we tell ourselves." It means that humans have the unique ability to create their own version of reality based on what our brains tell us. And often these stories are not good or healthy for us in terms of self-esteem and self-confidence. They disconnect us from remembering and harnessing our strengths and abilities.

One of the characters I see people play in their stories is that of "The Doubter," a term I first heard in Marcia Wieder's book *Dream, Clarify, and Create.*[16] Wieder is the founder of the Meaning Institute, where she teaches people to create and live fulfilling lives. The Doubter is that internal character that always brings up a huge list of concerns and issues that only serve to hold you back. The Doubter loves to limit your beliefs in yourself. Wieder notes that if you ignore The Doubter, it just gets louder and louder, and soon it takes over your reality, and your goals and dreams are smothered.

Wieder explains that The Doubter voice is often heard saying such things as, "I don't think that's a good idea." It might even say bold things such as, "Are you out of your mind?" The only reason to listen to The Doubter (before you turn the volume down) is because that voice can help you identify your limiting beliefs, which is a huge obstacle for most people. Haven't you ever heard a friend say something like, "I'd like to apply for that new special project or job that opened at work, but I doubt if my boss thinks I have the right skill set for it. Or would recommend me." And don't you just want to shake some sense into them for that self-sabotaging thought? You know they are more than qualified. Why don't they realize it?

The voice of The Doubter typically says things like, "I've tried before, and it didn't work out. I'm not going to do it again." Or "I got passed over again for a promotion; I must not be good enough." Limiting beliefs like this is a sign that you are operating in brain-off mode because you are falling prey to negative and unrealistic thinking and sabotaging your strengths.

BRAIN CHECK: Limiting beliefs are a problem because they are hard to identify. It's like white noise in your head, canceling out your self-confidence and your dreams and aspirations. Take two minutes and write down some limiting beliefs you have told yourself over the last day or week. Your answers might sound like some of these:

- No matter how hard I try, I'll never make it.
- It's too late to do something new.
- I'm too old.
- I'm too busy.
- I don't deserve it.
- I can't buy into this
- I don't have a choice.

LIMITING BELIEFS

_____

_____

_____

Circle the ones you tend to say a lot or that bring up the strongest reaction in your body as you read through them. Remind your brain that these beliefs aren't helpful and are costing you a lot. Let your brain know it's time to switch to the thinking-and-wise mode. It's time to loosen the grip these beliefs have on you. Take your limiting beliefs and write a new statement with a more positive one.

LIMITING BELIEFS, REWRITTEN

_____

_____

_____

SOCIAL SABOTAGE

Most of us work or communicate with other people during the day, so it's critical to understand the circumstance when unpleasant or unhealthy social interactions take your brain offline and deplete your energy. Social saboteurs can prevent us from having the energy to maximize our strengths and have an Energizer state during the day. When you encounter any social obstacles, it's like an immediate power outage. Depending on the situation, it can lead to a downward spiral of low confidence, low self-esteem, and feeling unappreciated.

Peer pressure is a negative influencer that can throw us into brain-off mode and derail us from using our strengths during the day. Joining a project that you aren't interested in, saying yes to every request, and believing office gossip are just a couple of social saboteurs that can take your brain offline. Since we spend so much of our day at work interacting with people, it's important to understand how your threat-and-reward system impacts your social encounters at work. Remember, we run away from anything threatening, and we walk toward anything we perceiving as rewarding.

Dr. David Rock, author of *Your Brain at Work* and founder of the NeuroLeadership Institute, created a model called SCARF to identify the five domains of social threats and rewards. These "social threats" can activate our brain's survival system like actual physical threats. People become the T-Rexes and saber-toothed tigers at work, and they easily flip our thinking brain off and our emotional brain on. As we've learned, once our brain goes offline, so does the access to the energy that fuels a day of using our strengths. I think it's important for everyone to assess your SCARFs. Because I work with people all day, I use this model all the time (at least three to five times a day at work) to understand why my brain went offline in a social situation. It helps to explain the strong emotional reactions we have to social situations (digital or in person), and why it's often so hard to control them. It also helps me understand why I start doubting myself (and how my limiting beliefs instantly override and prevent me from using my gifts and strengths). It's our instincts at work (literally!), and we need to be aware when to change them, to be back in Brain On! mode and aligned with our unique strengths and abilities.

The SCARF Model is based on the threats and rewards around the domains of Status, Certainty, Autonomy, Relatedness, and Fairness:

STATUS is about relative importance to others, or a perception of where we are in relation to the people around us. For example, if you were not invited to a meeting related to a project you were working on or didn't receive an email that everyone else on your team did, your brain might perceive it as a threat to your status and instantly go into brain-off mode. This may lead you to question your value, your abilities, your contribution to the team or organization.

CERTAINTY is about eliminating ambiguity. The brain is a pattern-recognition machine that is constantly trying to make accurate predictions of the near future to ensure our survival, so it craves certainty. It naturally wants to try and make sense out of the unfamiliar. In today's world, there is little certainty. On top of that, at work little things can create uncertainty, such as being unclear of expectations, requirements of an assignment, deadlines, your new customer's needs, and if that person's scowl during a meeting was because of something you said or did. Our threat systems are on high alert, and it's often due to uncertainty. If this switch is flipped to brain-off mode, you don't have access to your strengths to help you problem solve and focus on what you can control.

AUTONOMY is the perception of having control over our environment, a feeling of having choices and opportunities to focus on what we are good at. Our inability to influence outcomes triggers our threat sensors, which results in a fight-or-flight response.

RELATEDNESS involves deciding whether we are "in" or "out" of a particular social group. People naturally like to form their "community," so they experience a sense of belonging at work. If you feel isolated based on your role or excluded from a meeting, an important client email, or project, your threat response may include subjecting yourself to peer pressure to get back with the "in crowd." Or in good standing with your leadership. You may say yes to projects or requests that you don't have time for and don't align to your core strengths or interests.

FAIRNESS is knowing that you are being treated consistently with your peers. This goes beyond the big issues around pay equity or gender equity or social justice issues at a workplace. I want you to be aware of the daily types of interactions when our brains are threatened and perceive a threat of something not being fair. Why did that person get invited, not me? Why am I given that task, not someone else? Why was that person's work praised in a meeting and not that big project I just worked on? You can see how this threat response can be a subtle but energy-zapping saboteur and silently turn your wise brain off a lot during the day.

Engaged employees experience high levels of positive reward in the SCARF domains, whereas disengaged employees experience high levels of threats in these domains. We each tend to have one or two of these threat categories that are more dominant for us.

I find Uncertainty is one of my top SCARF threats. When I'm triggered at work, it's mainly because I don't understand something I'm expected to do or that it involves my participation. To be Brain On! again, I've adopted the saying, "Not to spoil the ending, but everything will be fine." I'm practicing getting comfortable with uncertainty all the time. This quote hangs on my office wall as a constant reminder.

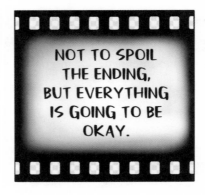

My second-highest SCARF threat is Autonomy. I have learned based on my purpose (Inspire, Create, and Innovate) and having one of my CliftonStrengths being a Futurist, that I really need autonomy over my work projects to focus on being creative and developing new ideas. When I feel my autonomy is threatened, like being required to attend an all-day mandatory training or working full-time in an office, my brain shuts down. That is just how I'm wired. I need to perform mental well-being exercises (you will learn more about them in Part Two) to stay Brain On! during those times when autonomy isn't possible. But I know for me to fully use my strengths, this is a key requirement and motivator for having an Energizing workday.

> BRAIN CHECK Take a moment to review the last day or week. Using the SCARF model, what situations created a threat or reward response in you? Which two domains are more dominant for you?

PART ONE HIGHLIGHT REEL

You've already learned a lot about how our brains work and how that knowledge can help you stay Brain On! Here is a summary of highlights from Part One:

- Our brains haven't had an "upgrade" since the beginning of time. They still function primarily as they did for our ancestors who walked the earth thousands of years ago.

Like our cave-dwelling ancestors, your brain is designed mainly to *keep you safe*, not to *keep you happy*.

- Your brain is always thinking: reward or threat? Your brain's primary organizing system is to sort every input or stimulus into two buckets: threat or reward. That means our brain's default is to consider everything as either 1) potentially causing harm or even death, or 2) being an innocent and safe interaction for us.

- Your brain's amygdala is what trips you up. Our prefrontal cortex is always competing with the emotional center of our brain and especially the amygdala. This part of the brain elicits our emotional responses. In today's complex world, our amygdala is on hyperalert and responding in that fight-flight-freeze routine. Over and over, all day long. Wearing our energy down until we feel edgy and unhappy.

- Our amygdala is always scanning and reacting to obstacles. There it goes again, getting us sidetracked by all kinds of emotional and psychological obstacles and distractions during the day. Dealing with these challenges and distractions can take up more than 50 percent of your day.

- Your job is to help your brain manage these inner and outer obstacles. We need to train our brain to be aware of when the "threat" or alarm system is going off and make sure the wiser, thinking part of the brain is on for healthier responses. When you manage the inner obstacles first, this will lead to successful management of the external ones.

- It takes a lot of our body's energy to run our brain. Most of this energy is wasted on negative thinking and fear-based responses, especially on responses based on your default mode of survival—ready to fight, flee, or freeze.

- Strive to be in Energizer mode. This is when you are Brain On! and feeling the highest level of energy and focus. You accomplish more, find more meaning in your day, feel a sense of belonging and connectedness, and can spend more time on goals you want to achieve.

We're at the end of Part One—hopefully you've gained awareness and insights into how your brain works, as well as why you have control over your happiness and success at work. Next up is Part Two — my Brain On! Individual Daily Playbook where you'll learn my top mental fitness techniques and well-being tips to start to train your brain to stay energized and support you in being your best at work, starting now.

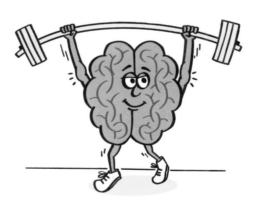

PART TWO

BRAIN ON! INDIVIDUAL DAILY PLAYBOOK

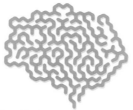

Remember that I called myself your mental fitness trainer at the beginning of the book? I take my job very seriously in helping you improve your mental fitness at work. We've never been taught to focus on our mental fitness before. That is one reason I'm writing this book. Improving your mental fitness will ensure you reach Energizer mode, which is critical to achieving a higher level of well-being and accomplishing your goals at work. Why does this matter? Many workplaces today measure an individual's success as "meeting or exceeding" expectations based on whether you achieved **what** you set out to do. But the key to your well-being and being in an Energizer mode depends on not only what you achieved, but also on **how** you achieved it. That is the Brain On! difference. Were you stressed out all the time to get to your goal? Did you like the skills and tasks associated with that goal? Did it re-energize you every time you worked on it? Did you learn something new that you enjoyed?

It's time to upgrade how we set goals at work based on how energized we feel by them. In this next part of the book, I'm really in my trainer glory to help you determine your goals in new ways and ensure that you achieve them in a positive, energy-sustaining, and mentally healthy way. Picture me with power trainers on, a baseball cap (with a cool Brain On! logo), and a thick clipboard in my hand. We are going to learn some mental fitness warm-up exercises and daily strategies to keep your brain in Energizer mode every day on the playing field (aka work).

The Brain On! Individual Daily Playbook is a fresh and easy approach to managing your workday. It puts your thinking brain in the driver's seat to accomplish your goals and avoid those nasty speed bumps and potholes that can throw your day off. You are going to learn to attain and maintain an Energizer state by making better moment-by-moment choices. Just like in a real sports game, it's the split-second decisions that often determine a successful outcome in the end.

Ready?
Let's go!

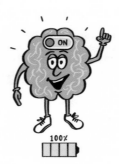

CHAPTER 5

THE NEW STRENGTHS-BASED WORK GOALS

"Where should I focus my energy?"

I f you were working with a fitness trainer at the gym, the two of you would agree on specific goals, such as increased endurance, weight loss, greater strength, or more flexibility. You might want to lose weight for health reasons, increase your endurance to be more active outdoors, become stronger so you don't get sore working out or working in the yard, or gain flexibility to counteract sitting at a desk most of the day.

Any kind of physical training goal is attained by committing to daily exercises over time—you don't build stronger arm muscles or lose ten pounds in a week. Think of how a professional Ironman tri-athlete is devoted to their training. Their long-term goal is competing in and winning a grueling 140.6-mile competition. They need to stay focused on maximizing their key strengths (sound familiar?) while performing their "work" job of swimming, biking, and running. Their eight-hour "workday" is committed to specific training routines to build endurance. These athletes dedicate significant time working up to their peak performance.

Having a goal of competing in, much less winning, an Ironman Triathlon is one that few of us will ever have. But the same principles apply to setting goals in your own workday and keeping in peak mental shape to achieve them. Your primary mental fitness goal is to achieve and stay in Energizer mode, so you have the brain power and motivation to achieve your strengths-based goals in the workplace. Goals are your GPS for the workday, and they give your brain a positive and more evolved focus instead of constantly getting distracted and continuously scanning for threats in its primal mode.

I know that the word "goal" can sometimes throw a brain offline because it may bring up negative emotions and disappointment about goals that weren't reached in the past, or ones that someone else set for us. Keep the more neutral dictionary definition of a goal in front of you— "the end toward which effort is directed" —to remind yourself that it is all about focusing your energy. The key word here being focus. Setting goals is a foundational mental skill that trains your brain to focus on what you want and where you want to go. Doesn't that make perfect sense? Your time is a precious resource. Why apply your valuable brain energy to something you don't want or care about?

Goal is that four-letter word that can seem more daunting than climbing Mount Everest if not put into context and you aren't excited about it. A fitness trainer in the gym would never give you the goal of pressing one hundred pounds in a month if you can't press ten pounds right now. When I talk about goals, I'm not talking about those "go big or go home" ones. As high achievers, we're all programmed to set big, hairy, audacious goals. Big goals can be more burdensome than they are motivational. They seem more daunting to accomplish and sustain from day to day. It's great to dream big, but the Brain On! way to *achieve* something big is to start small.

Goal-Setting Exercise

Think back to something you accomplished at work that was rewarding, energizing, and brought you true joy. Was it developing a new training class? Did you mentor a new colleague? Were you assigned the lead on a mission-critical project? Did you complete a difficult assignment not only on time, but better than you or your manager hoped? This type of reflection exercise is extremely helpful in developing new goals. It helps prime your brain to get creative and energized and brings in your strengths to incorporate the next time.

LET'S TRY IT: Write down a couple of these work experiences you've had. How could you use these experiences as a template for replicating motivating and engaging goals?

An energizing goal I recently accomplished at work:

_____

_____

_____

Knowing your goals and acting on them are the "secret sauce" to keeping you motivated and achieving the Energizer state day in and day out. But these goals will be most meaningful to you if they aligned to your strengths. Focusing on aligning our strengths with our goals is something we aren't taught and don't take time to do.

This chapter and its exercises are designed to help you identify, create, and evaluate goals that will maximize your Energizer state and lead to a higher level of satisfaction at work—the feeling that you've contributed to the organization with your own unique skills. Instead of setting goals solely based on your company's objectives, standard job descriptions, or performance review checklists, we're going to flip the script and create work goals for you that are tailored to your own personal strengths. Identifying your strengths and applying them to your goals is a new way of approaching work. Your goals are aligned to your natural talents and stretches them a bit, which produces more fulfilling and joyful days at work.

Why is it important to set goals with your strengths in mind? Because according to Gallup, goals "too often are intended to punish ourselves for 'poor' behavior, for a talent we don't have, or for an accomplishment we haven't achieved."[17] There's a big difference between "need to do goals" and "growth goals." Our brains have been trained to set goals based on tasks instead of what is meaningful and will improve our work life. Gallup reminds us that strengths-based goals allow you to take those work objectives you want to focus on or have been asked to focus on and incorporate your needs and natural talents as well by focusing on:

- What's important to you.
- How you want to grow.
- What changes you want to see.
- What talents you can use to achieve the goals.

Short- and Long-Term Goal Setting

First, we're going to create a list of both short- and long-term goals. These should always be top of mind each day, as they serve as your personal GPS guides at work (and also in life). You want to think of goals that will lead to you:

- Feeling energized, calm, hopeful, joyful.
- Creating a full battery at the end of day.
- Developing stronger connections and relationships.
- Ensuring you did meaningful work.
- Contributing to something bigger than yourself.
- Feeling valued and recognized.

When you make these two lists, use whatever method you normally do to create your goals with your manager or team leader. Consider short-term goals as something to achieve in the next month. Long-term goals may stretch out to a year or more. And remember, they can still be a compilation of small goals. They don't have to take deep thought and a lot of time and be some grandiose vision. Write down as many as you can think of. Then go back and choose a couple that get you most excited about how you want to spend your time at work in the coming weeks or months.

SHORT-TERM GOALS:

_____

_____

_____

LONG-TERM GOALS:

_____

_____

_____

Let's do a final check on the list of goals you created above to make sure they are goals that are meaningful, attainable, and will lead to a happier, healthier, Energizer workday. The goals should:

Align with your values—focus your goals on the things that matter most to you.

Defined clearly—you should be able to clearly note when you've reached each step.

Easily ownable—make sure you truly want what you're working toward to make the goal your own.

Realistic yet challenging—be sure that your goals are achievable within a reasonable amount of time yet challenge you to grow.

Positively framed—state your goals in positive terms that will result in a more fulfilling feeling when accomplished.

Be SMART—goals are Specific, Measurable, Achievable, Realistic, and Time-bound.

New Way of Setting Goals

Now we are going to look at these goals in the new Brain On! way by adding your strengths so you can maximize your natural talents and stay energized at work.

Let's revisit your three-word strength assessment from Chapter 4. It's critical to keep your strengths front and center as you set your goals for the day, week, and month ahead.

Rewrite your three strengths here:

_____

_____

_____

We're going to make your goals SMART-ER by first adding these strengths. Some positive psychologists like to think of the E as standing for Evaluative and Ethical. I like to think of it as Execution—are you pursuing the goal in a way that results in a healthy outcome for you? It's about not just *what* you achieved, but *how* you achieved it.

There's no sense pursuing a work goal that leaves you burning the midnight oil, grabbing unhealthy snacks to get you through, or becoming highly anxious, stressed, and even sick. You won't do your best work because your brain is not in the Energizer state.

The R in SMART-ER refers to Rewarding and in a positive and intrinsic motivational sense, not purely a financial or external reward. Ensuring a goal is intrinsically motivating and rewarding is the key to keeping you Brain On! and focused.

Strengths-Based Goal-Setting Exercise

We're going to take your list of short- and long-term goals you just made, and then rewrite them to include your strengths. If you need to take a break here for five minutes, please do so. I want you to be Brain On! as I'm going to walk you through how I did this exercise for myself so you can see how this is done.

DEB'S STRENGTHS-BASED GOAL-SETTING EXAMPLE

I first came up with four basic goals for the coming year:

1. Develop the requirements and specifications to upgrade PEQ (a well-being product I created that we sell, implement, and service).

2. Deliver my final book manuscript to the publisher by June 1.

3. Increase our well-being and engagement brand awareness.

4. Create a strategic plan for integrating our well-being solutions into all new lines of business.

Next, after reviewing the list, I've been trained and taught (as have almost all of us) to make sure the goals are SMART. So, goals 1, 3, and 4 from above are missing some of these elements and can be refined. The changes are shown in blue below as I update my original goals 1, 3, and 4 to make them SMART:

1.   Develop the requirements and specifications to upgrade PEQ by October 1.

2.   Deliver my final book manuscript to the publisher by June 1.

3.   Increase our well-being and engagement brand awareness by getting three articles in two major trade publications by September 1.

4.   Create a strategic plan for integrating our well-being solutions into all new lines of business by August 1.

But what I found over the years is that by stopping here, and only using SMART goals, it can derail us from really achieving and focusing on our goals every day. To ensure we continue to stay focused and inspired (and not get burned out, frustrated, disengaged, and brain off), we need to incorporate our strengths to achieve these goals. So, I wove my strengths into these statements, shown below in pink. It's helpful if you use verbs and action words, as your strengths are what will help intrinsically motivate you to take the right action.

I will use my creativity to

I will apply my futuristic lens to

I will tap into my strengths of building connections to

Now, here are my updated goals 1-4 that incorporate my strengths and their impact, shown in pink:

1. Using my creative talents, I will develop unique requirements and specifications to upgrade PEQ that will differentiate us from our competition by October 1.

2. Harnessing my project management abilities, I will deliver my final book manuscript to the publisher by June 1.

3. Increase our well-being and engagement brand awareness by tapping into my innovative and futuristic strengths to secure three articles in two major trade publications by September 1.

4. Create a strategic plan for integrating our well-being solutions into all new lines of business by capitalizing on my networking and ideation skills by August 1.

Now that we've added our strengths, the final step is to ensure these strengths-based goals are SMART-ER by incorporating *how* we achieve them. I suggest adding to each goal the well-being qualities and characteristics you want to maintain that will allow you to achieve your goals in the healthiest, most productive, and energizing way. Something that will also help guide you as you dive into the details of your goals and ensure you measure not only what milestones you are accomplishing, but how you are accomplishing them. Creating a new, high-quality product by the deadline is one thing, but if you also ended up going to the hospital with panic attacks or high blood pressure, or your relationship fell apart because you were working too hard, to me (and probably to you as well) you really didn't successfully achieve that goal.

Add modifiers to your goal statements such as while, at the same time, during this time, throughout this time, and the whole time. Let's apply some examples using these modifiers:

- While checking in a couple of times throughout the day to make sure I'm in Energizer state, and Brain On!
- While also maintaining a healthy relationship with my family.
- And disconnecting during the evenings and weekends.
- And feeling excited and not stressed out. Enjoying the project even during challenging times.
- While monitoring my stress level to ensure I don't get burned out or exhausted at the end of the day.
- Managing on one cup of caffeine a day and looking for healthy ways to maintain my energy levels.
- Taking breaks every two hours while working on the project.
- Disconnect on the weekends to recharge and re-energize.
- Get adequate sleep during the busy cycles.
- Attending family events, games, and school programs.
- Building strong, positive connections with my team.
- Staying on schedule with my daily walks and exercise routine.
- During which time I'm aware of and regulating my emotions.

So here are my final goal statements revised to be SMART-ER, showing not just what I'm going to accomplish but *how* I'm going to, shown in yellow:

1. Using my creative talents, I will develop unique requirements and specifications to upgrade PEQ that will differentiate us

from our competition **by October 1** while creating a virtual working environment to foster collaboration and community.

2. Harnessing my project management abilities, I will **deliver my final book manuscript to the publisher by June 1** while ensuring I remain Brain On!, have fun, and celebrate small wins during the writing process.

3. Increase our well-being and engagement brand awareness by tapping into my innovative and futuristic strengths **to secure three articles in two major trade publications by September 1,** while ensuring I build in rest and recovery time.

4. Create a strategic plan for integrating our well-being solutions into all new lines of business by capitalizing on my networking and ideation skills **by August 1.** The plan will incorporate realistic deadlines, a schedule of priorities, and my health objectives to help ensure I don't get burned out trying to complete everything in a short period of time.

Now it's your turn! Start with some of the goals you wrote earlier in this chapter (either short or long term) and rewrite them using the SMART-ER approach by weaving in your strengths and well-being qualities you'll use to accomplish them.

Your SMART-ER Goals

SMART-ER GOAL 1

_____

_____

_____

SMART-ER GOAL 2

_____

_____

_____

Trainer Tips: Achieving Your Goals

You've set the foundation for an Energizer workday with strengths-based SMART-ER goals. Before we cover the strategies to remain in Energizer mode during the daily obstacle course, here are a few of my favorite and proven tips on always keeping your goals front and center:

TIP 1: GOALS HAPPEN THROUGH DAILY HABITS

You've spent some time thinking about your goals and committing them to paper. You've got a destination in mind. The results you want to achieve by a certain date. But a goal that is not made a priority and acted upon each day is just a wish or a hope.

In his bestselling book *Atomic Habits: Tiny Changes, Remarkable Results*, James Clear delves deeper into supporting goals through a specific process or system. He explains that goals are the results, while systems are the processes that lead to the result. He explains the "system" is your journey of daily small habits that get you closer and closer to your desired outcome. It's the daily habits that inspire motivation and lead to self-improvement. Habits are the repeated behaviors we commit to doing each day that will systematically help us achieve our goal. It's okay if you have a couple of days or weeks where you are recharging your batteries, but when too many days go by and you don't prioritize habits leading to a goal, it's easy to never achieve it, and we're left wondering where all the time went.

So why is it so hard to prioritize good habits that will lead to goal attainment? It goes back to that reptilian brain of ours, the part that is designed to save as much energy as possible to keep the body safe. That's why we can't rely on willpower alone to make healthy changes, as our brain will always default to a brain-off, threat-based response. You need to develop habits that will stick. And this starts with a daily planning session.

TIP 2: GET STARTED IN THE MORNING WITH A CLEAR PLAN

Going back to the sport analogy, a team wouldn't go out onto the field without a game plan. The game would result in chaos and probably a loss. Same goes for your day and working toward your goal—without a clear plan you are setting yourself up for failure. As James Clear notes, "stop waiting for motivation or inspiration to strike you and set a schedule for your habits." The message here is clear (pardon the pun): Motivation flows from action, not the other way around.

Put your goals into action by planning out those daily tasks and habits that will deliver meaningful progress. First, make sure you don't have too many goals you're working on at once, either short term or long term. Look at your workweek overall as a whole. There's only so many hours in the week, and decide which goals make sense to work on daily, while others just a couple of times that week.

Try to conduct your daily planning session at the same time every day, preferably early in the morning. Bundle this new habit with another habit you do every morning, like drinking coffee or sitting on the train into work. Creating a plan each morning should only take five minutes or so. It helps to do it the same time each day. For me, I do it at 7:30 a.m. over a cup of coffee. I set a "soothing" alarm on my phone as a reminder in case I get distracted by a news story or a call from my kids.

TIP 3: TWEAK YOUR PLAN WHEN NECESSARY

You've made planning your day a habit, translated your strengths-based goals into actionable tasks, and found a way to prioritize what needs to be done each day. However, don't let your brain run on autopilot. Take some time occasionally to review whether your approach to daily planning is helping you move toward your goal and keeping your brain in Energizer mode.

- Are my days calm and intentional or stressful and haphazard?
- Did I complete all my daily planning sessions or skip some?
- Do I feel accomplished at the end of most days?
- Are my high priority tasks being addressed?
- Am I on track to meet my long-term goals?
- This day was especially productive — why?
- I accomplished nothing impactful on this day — why?
- Have I played to my strengths?

That last question is the most important one of all. When you find a couple of hours a day to engage in applying your strengths to projects, instead of just ticking off a to-do list efficiently and automatically, you'll truly be more joyful and engaged at work.

TIP 4: VISUALIZE YOUR GOALS

Have you ever heard the phrase, "What you focus on grows?" If you focus on problems, your brain will find more problems. If you focus on your goals, you achieve those goals. So, in addition to incorporating goals into your daily plan, another way you achieve your goals is to visualize being successful. Visualization is the technique when you mentally imagine yourself performing your projects or tasks exactly how you would like them to occur in real life. It's like a mental rehearsal. The basic concept is that when you consistently rehearse your meetings, presentations, or tasks in your mind, you will improve the actual performance of them. If you have trouble with mental visualization, try using verbal affirmations instead.

TIP 5: COMMIT TO IT OR DUMP IT

Are there goals you've had for years and haven't started? Some of us have had lifelong dreams or goals year after year that continuously plague us because we think about them but don't act. Every time we think about them or write them down and don't act on them our brain equates that to incomplete or failure and that file card gets stored in our memory. It's time to decide: Do it or Dump it. If you choose to write a goal down, commit to it. Take action every day to make it happen. Otherwise, it's time for a new goal or dream.

GREAT JOB! We're at the end of goal-setting warmup exercises and tips, and now you're ready to tackle the day! But wait, if you remember from Chapter 2, we know that unexpected internal and external obstacles are just going to be part of our day. Take a deep breath—I'm going to give you my Six Strategies to stay in an Energizer state and prevent these obstacles from getting in the way of achieving your goals and winning your workday.

CHAPTER 6
SIX STRATEGIES FOR AN ENERGIZER DAY

"How do I overcome daily obstacles?"

Every day is going to have some obstacles no matter how well we've planned it or tried to anticipate what is on the horizon. Knowing and accepting this fact goes a long way in not beating yourself up when your brain starts to go offline, and you feel its energy depleting. Think about a day sometime in the last few weeks when things didn't go so well, and you felt like you achieved nothing of significance:

- What specifically went wrong?
- What goals were not met?
- What obstacle prevented you from being in an Energizer state?

My wish for you after reading this chapter is that you start to see how you can create more high-performance workdays and fewer days when obstacles wore you down or tripped you up.

My family would tell you I'm not known for my cooking (I can barely "make" ice, and I burn water), but I am an expert on the recipe and ingredients for a Brain On! workday. You've learned that from the minute you wake up, your brain's energy will only start to decrease. Your job is to maintain your brain's power for as long as possible throughout the day, so that you end your day in that Energizer state and possibly even more energized than you started. Imagine that!

I'm going to walk you through managing your daily obstacle course and show you how to stay on track throughout your day to find more joy, energy, productivity, and even fun. Think of this chapter as now being "on the field," and you've got to stay on your toes (or in this case, Brain On!) to run around or through the "blockers" that get in the way of you reaching your goals for the day.

Avoiding the inevitable obstacles each day is what will keep you in an Energizer state which is your ultimate and overarching goal at work each day. Here are my Six Strategies to get you there:

1. Start with a success mindset.
2. Set an intention for good.
3. Tackle hard things first.
4. Build in breaks.
5. Insert motivation.
6. Check in with yourself.

Start with a Success Mindset

No team goes out onto the field thinking it's going to be a losing battle. But we can easily put ourselves into that mindset by veering from our daily plan by checking our work emails before getting out of bed or letting our inner voice take us immediately to a fearful or negative place when we first open our eyes.

High-performing people don't leave their mindset up to chance. They actively work to overcome any misguided thoughts, poor emotional regulation, and irrational (primal) fears. That's why training your brain is as important as aerobic conditioning to lead a healthy life.

Starting your day with a successful mindset begins by avoiding your phone, your calendar, or anything that throws you into a work mode very first thing when you awake. Your brain needs time to get online in a positive and energizing way.

Here are some ways you can prep for an energizing day:

- **Don't trigger your brain's alarm with your phone's alarm.** Turning off a phone alarm requires you physically picking up your phone. Once it is in your hand, it's going to be difficult to put it down again. You'll start checking emails, social media, texts, and off you go to the work races without being mentally prepared. No matter how pleasant of an alarm sound you think you've chosen, it's likely not as gentle as the sounds and sights of nature. Many well-being experts, including myself, suggest that alarms that emulate natural elements such as rainfall or a bird chirping or even alarms that mimic the rising sun are best.

The goal is not to immediately zap your brain power and hijack your amygdala with the first sounds of the morning. Rather choose a device to wake you up gently.

- **Monitor your news and social media intake.** Digesting this type of information can be toxic pollution for your brain, especially first thing in the morning. News stories can start to trigger a flood of negative emotions and throw your brain offline in a big way. Positive psychology researchers Shawn Achor and Michelle Gielan report[18] that people who watch just three minutes of negative news in the morning have a whopping 27 percent greater likelihood of reporting their day as unhappy later in the day. Achor also notes that watching negative news can diminish work productivity. Our goal in the morning is to prime our day to be a good one. Don't let negative news influence your brain's start to the day. Starting the day with optimism will help your brain see the possibilities instead of the problems.

- **Center yourself.** What is a morning routine without news, emails, and texting? A healthy morning routine is one that gives you a sense of calm, appreciation, and perspective. Choose something restorative that you like—inspirational reading, writing in a journal, doing a gratitude practice, or gentle yoga or stretching. Connecting to a deeper and more meaningful place inside yourself first thing in the morning will help you stay centered throughout the day.

- **Consciously start your workday.** Don't just slide into it. Decide exactly when your brain is officially "on-the-job" and focused on work. Will it start on your commute with phone calls to a client or your team? Setting up your day for success starts with how you show up and what you do first. This sets the tone for the rest of your day, so it's important to build a habit of consciously saying "Brain On!" Check in to make sure you are consciously paying attention to your brain being activated as you start the workday. A great cue and habit is to say to yourself as you power on your computer or work equipment and start your day, "Power On! Brain On!" This kind of mantra helps you consciously turn on your thinking brain.

Set an Intention for Good

Your brain is probably asking right now, "what's the difference between a goal and an intention?" Good question. An intention is the attitude you want to cultivate throughout the day. It's the feeling you want to maintain as you move through the day. A goal is a specific end point or result you want to achieve.

Your intention can be something like, "I am grounded," or "I am joyous," or "I am courageous." Your intention should only take a few seconds to calibrate. It's like hitting the "start" on your GPS system—you want to start out on the right foot mentally to get there. My intentions tend to focus around three themes: Be kind, Be of service, and Have fun! One leader I work with told me he tends to get off track the minute he sets foot in the office. His intentions are Stay focused and Stay connected.

It can also be very helpful to set an intention before each meeting or a chunk of work you are about to start. And especially before a very important meeting or a big phone call. Ask yourself questions such as "how do I want to show up in this meeting?" Or "how do I want to feel during this difficult conversation?" Take a close look at what your motivations are as you set your intentions—wouldn't it be more satisfying to be a force for good in the world?

Tackle Hard Things First

We touched upon this briefly in Chapter 5, but as you are planning your day, prioritize working on the most important goal you want to make progress on that day. For most of us, our mental energy tends to be highest in the morning. But if you feel most energized and clear-headed midday or late in the day, go with that. The point is science has proven you only have about three to four hours of productive "brain power" and resources each day, and that's about it. And you need to strategically protect and use that time and space to make progress on the more complex, creative, and high-priority and strategic projects, including your goals for the day. Not only will that help you complete that important item, but it will also give you an "accomplishment high" for the entire day. That, in turn, infuses your mood, which helps sustain your energy and allows you to be more productive and resilient all day—it's a virtuous cycle.

To start, define what your "prime working time" really is. I have a client who runs international markets for a large hedge fund. He gets up at 3:30 a.m. most days to speak with customers abroad. That early time is not "his morning." He gets to his office by 6:30 a.m.—that's his morning. He goes into a conference room, closes the door, performs an easy stretching routine, meditates for five minutes, and then pulls out his notebook to write down his one "must win" for the day. Then he goes to his desk and immediately starts working on his "must win." He's usually interrupted within thirty or forty minutes, but by then he has made some progress and knows how he will handle what he needs to. His routine helps him gain perspective and set his intention so that even amidst the chaos of the day he can focus on what's important.

I have another client, a philanthropist, who sits on three public company boards and four nonprofit boards. She gets up at 7 a.m. every morning and makes an espresso. She sits on her porch to write in her journal for twenty minutes, then she goes for a long walk in the woods by her home. When she returns, she focuses on projects that are long term and strategic for her organizations or her life. By the time her phone starts ringing or the emails start coming, she has already made progress.

Your morning and your life will look different, so you need to tailor your routine to work for you. Define the time that works best for you to focus on your goals, then decide what you will do with it, with the intention of proactively giving yourself a calm and nourishing start and making progress on something that matters.

Build in Breaks

Think of your daily course at work as broken up into mini-sprints—you perform a task, recover, and then transition to the next task. These mini-sprints happen several times a day or more depending on your workload or responsibilities. The recovery period is your break period, and you are not being a slacker or lazy in taking several throughout the day.

There is actual scientific evidence on why people should take periodic breaks at work. Breaks keep us from getting bored and unfocused. When you're in the groove of a task or project, the ideas are flowing, and you feel great. But it doesn't last forever—stretch yourself just a bit beyond that productivity zone and you might feel unfocused, zoned out, or even irritable. As I mentioned early in this book, the human brain just wasn't built for the extended focus we ask of it these days. A short break is really all we need to get back on track.

Breaks also help us retain information better. Our brains have two modes: the "focused mode," which we use when we're doing things like learning something new, writing, or working, and "diffuse mode," which is our more relaxed, daydreamy mode when we're not thinking so hard. You might think that the focused mode is the one to optimize for more productivity, but diffuse mode is when we absorb information more deeply. The beauty of taking a break is that it allows us to step back and make sure we're accomplishing the right things and in the right way. When you work on a task continuously, it's easy to lose focus and get lost in the weeds. Taking a break is a great habit (and one not to feel guilty about) because it encourages us to stay mindful of our goals.

BRAIN CHECK: One important element that Tony Schwartz, a well-known American journalist and founder of the Energy Project, emphasizes is that all breaks are not created equal. That is, a break only counts (meaning it's restorative and energizing) if during that time you do something you enjoy or that is renewing for you. Doom scrolling doesn't count.

It's not regenerating. To take advantage of any break, it's important to avoid the pitfall of going into autopilot mode. We are creatures of habit and often we run for our phones, junk food, or a mindless website during our free time. Schwartz, author of *The Way We Work Isn't Working*,[19] recommends developing a break cheat sheet. This is a mental fitness exercise that basically outlines what activities you like to do when you have a one-minute, five-minute or even ten-minute break that will boost your mood and re-energize you. For example, my break cheat sheet includes the following:

ONE MINUTE

- Three deep breaths.
- Stand up and stretch.
- Look out the window at nature.
- Read a funny joke.
- Take a couple sips of water or your favorite tea.
- Visualize your happy place or a beautiful nature scene.

FIVE MINUTES

- Go for a short walk.
- Listen to music.
- Play your favorite guided meditation.
- Fill up your water bottle.
- Bond with your pet or child (if they are around).

TEN MINUTES

- Get outside in nature.
- Do a ten-minute workout routine.

- Read a couple pages from your favorite novel.
- Call up a friend and say hi.
- Watch a couple of inspiring or funny videos (positive endorphins).

By having this laid out ahead of time, you are strategically ensuring a more successful, energizing break and making it an easy habit to implement.

Insert Motivation

You can proactively insert activities that will motivate you if you are having a lull in energy. For example, turn your attention to an activity you enjoy or—even better—an activity that will fill you with a sense of accomplishment or purpose. This is different from a break when you purposely disconnect completely from work. In this case, you may focus on similar types of activities, but with the specific goal of inspiring and energizing yourself. You planned out your day, but you can always rearrange it or insert an activity that focuses on your goals. Find a colleague at work you enjoy collaborating with and spend a few moments brainstorming with them. Call your partner or take a few deep breaths to regain perspective. Play music that energizes you. There is research on how listening to music, especially music designed for video games, can increase your productivity and motivation. Sometimes just getting back on plan is motivating. Or taking stock in what you've already accomplished so far can give you an extra push forward to tackle the rest. Life is distracting and fighting for focus is its own reward.

Check in with Yourself

This is the last strategy on the list, probably the most important, and the one that can be performed throughout your daily course. So many of our thoughts and actions are influenced by external and internal factors. The weather may put us in a good mood one moment. Conversely, you have a difficult conversation with a colleague, and you feel upset and depleted the next moment. Our moods change quickly and subconsciously and can be hard to control. When you step back and take notice of your moods and feelings throughout the day, it helps you reset your energy level. You can see more clearly why you are thinking and feeling a certain way, and this consciousness helps you deal with the ups and downs.

Self-awareness is key and the first step toward emotional regulation. If you don't check in with yourself, you don't know if you are brain off or Brain On! And before you know it, your day is over, and you're exhausted and totally stressed out. As your daily plan starts to take shape, it's important to build in a habit of check-ins with yourself. The reason we build them in here is so that you do them. Find three or four times that are consistent in your day-to-day schedule when you build in a Pause sign. Some natural Pause signs during the day are entering the office, going to the restroom, answering a text, during lunch, turning your computer on (is my Brain On?). Cues like this will help you build in these habits, so they become automatic.

Emotional check-ins are one of the most important things you can do for your mental well-being. They can instantly give you visibility into the stress and anxiety you may be feeling and the distractions you are experiencing. We're in such a rush to get to the next thing, or we want to avoid our negative emotions entirely, that we skip ahead past dealing with what we are feeling now. Emotional check-ins help you slow down. They're designed to help you get an accurate reading of how you feel. Taking an inventory of your feelings in the present moment will ensure you feel better in the future.

Think of these check-ins like the physical heart rate checks you do during an intense aerobic exercise session to see if you are "running" at a good, healthy pace or outside of your target zone (working too hard or not hard enough). Same thing applies here—trust me on this—you can't feel better *in an hour*, if you don't know how you feel *in the minute*. Here are five simple ways to do an emotional check-in.

- **Tune in to your body.** It sends physical signals about how you're feeling, long before your emotions fully register. Are your shoulders up in your ears and feeling tense, or is your heart racing superfast? These types of physical sensations are alerting you to your emotions needing some rebalancing.

- **Take a deep breath.** Slowing your breath down is one of the things you can do for your mental well-being. Breathe in through your nose and out through your mouth. When you slow your mind, you can focus on your emotional state of being.

- **Ask the one simple question.** "How am I feeling right in this moment?" This is a terrific mindfulness practice, and one that directs your attention to a very accurate reading of your emotional state.

- **Use vivid descriptions.** The more detailed and specific you can describe your feelings, the more helpful they can be. It's not helpful to tell yourself, "I feel bad." That is a vague comment. Try and get deeper into your feelings by using words such as hurt, rejected, overwhelmed, worried, judged, or exhausted. The more specific your description, the more specific you can be in knowing what you need to take care of yourself.

- **Reflect on what's causing the emotion.** It's often hard as humans to know why we are feeling something, as our lives and emotions aren't simple or easy. If you can reflect on what might be contributing to how you are feeling, it will give you the insight you need to manage your feelings and change your attitude.

Energizer Building Blocks

Congratulations! You've almost completed the Brain On! Individual Playbook! You are well on your way to becoming an expert at staying in the Energizer mode!

You may have broken some mental sweat working on your strengths-based goals (Building Block #1). Hopefully, you're starting to incorporate daily strategies, including creating positive intentions for how you show up each day at work and staying motivated with intrinsic rewards to keep you achieving your goals (Building Block #2).

Take note of the strengths-based goals you have identified and the changes you are making toward winning the workday. This is not a place to get down for what you have not yet mastered; this is a quick break to praise yourself for what you are doing better.

There are just two Building Blocks left to tackle—making nimble adjustments when your brain gets thrown offline during your day and giving yourself plenty of self-care to boost your brain's energy.

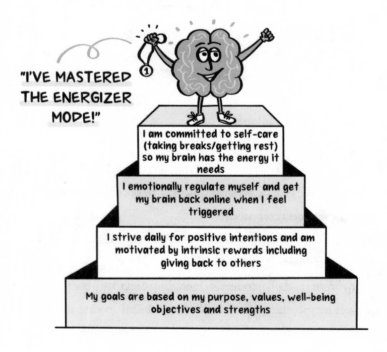

CHAPTER 7

BRAIN ON! MENTAL FITNESS EXERCISES

"How do I recover when I go offline?"

When people are asked about important relationships in life, they name the ones with their partner, their children, their parents, their siblings, their friends, and then boss or co-workers. No one would say their relationship with their brain is a top priority. But in the end, that is the most important relationship you will have. How we regulate our brain's responses and coach it into a healthy condition is what impacts these other relationships to be positive and fulfilling or negative and frustrating.

That's why I believe the Brain On! approach is revolutionary because it asks you to be aware of how your brain is functioning moment-by-moment, hour-by-hour each day. The old way of working is to grit your teeth through the stress and frustrations of the day, and then head home to flop on the couch or grab a drink to drown your anxiety at the local watering hole. The new Brain On! way is to check in on yourself throughout the day, to regulate your emotions or give your brain a break to maintain your energy and mood, and before you start your busy day, an important meeting, or a work session where you need to be highly focused and productive.

The primary function of your thinking brain at work is to keep you operating at optimal performance in your tasks, decisions, and interactions. You've already learned that your thinking brain and emotional brain can't be on at the same time. When your emotional brain goes into autopilot and overrides your thinking brain, it's difficult if not impossible to perform well at work. Performing exercises throughout the day to stay mentally strong allows you to say at the end of the day, *"I accomplished my goals and really took care of myself, too. I am ready to tackle tomorrow!"*

Your physical fitness regimen probably incorporates fundamentals such as weights, cardio, and flexibility exercises, that you then apply in real life playing golf and tennis, hiking on a trail, or distance biking. To keep mentally fit, you may be familiar with fundamental brain exercises such as guided meditation and mindfulness-based stress reduction. What I've found most helpful about mental fitness exercises is that I can use them to build my brain "muscles" throughout the workday. These mental fitness exercises help keep me Brain On! and operating at my best during the workday to handle those moments when I feel like I'm heading offline. I can easily call upon these practices to get back online in just a matter of minutes.

One of my favorite quotes and guiding North Stars in my life is from Ellen Langer, who is considered the "mother of mindfulness." She is a social psychologist and the first female professor to gain tenure in the Department of Psychology at Harvard University. Langer has penned more than eleven books, including her bestseller, *The Power of Mindful Learning.*[20]

Langer summarizes so simply and beautifully our true "job" in life, which is to manage our emotions moment by moment to create an energizing and Brain On! day:

"Life consists only of moments, nothing more than that.
So, if you make the moment matter, it all matters."

That's what this chapter is all about—simple and practical mental fitness exercises you can use in your day when you feel your brain is being thrown offline. I've included the most helpful and effective practices based on my years of working with individuals, as well as large and small employers, and hearing their positive feedback and success stories. While some of the mindfulness principles such as meditation and breathwork may not be new, I've tailored them to the work environment, so they require the minimum amount of time to perform but lead to maximum results.

Ready, Set, Power On!

As you learned in Chapter 6, having a Brain On! day at work starts by consciously telling your brain to Power On! just as you would power up your computer. Remind your brain that its task throughout the day is to stay in thinking mode and avoid being emotionally hijacked. One of the most effective mental fitness exercises I've discovered is the above the line/below the line concept devised by Jim Deth-mer, founding partner of The Conscious Leadership Group and co-author of *The 15 Commitments of Conscious Leadership: A New Paradigm for Sustainable Success,*[21] which creates these above/below questions to help locate your emotions in the present moment. It is a simple question to check in with yourself during the day to assess if you are Brain On! (above the line) or brain off (below the line).

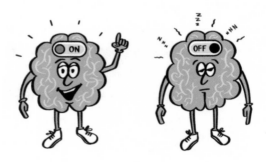

Above the line: Am I more interested in learning than in being right?

I am open in mind, emotions, and body.

I am curious and question my beliefs.

I listen to understand.

I am in a state of trust.

Below the line: Am I being defensive to prove I'm right?

I am in a state of threat.

I'm not listening; I'm feeling resentful.

I am closed to thoughts and emotions.

I am blaming.

When you start to feel overwhelmed, and your brain is falling off-line (and below the line), you can repeat one of the simple phrases below to calm down and get your brain back online. You can do this as you're walking down the hall, heating up your lunch, waiting to enter a virtual meeting, or walking around the block during a break. Say to yourself:

One moment at a time.

One task at a time.

One day at a time.

This too shall pass.

All is well.

I've got this.

What We're Avoiding: The Big Three Obstacles

Even when you are Brain On! and in Energizer mode, you can still unconsciously slip offline because of those pesky obstacles that pop up. Way back in chapter 2, you learned about internal and external obstacles and how they can sometimes make your day feel like a nonstop obstacle course. Staying aware of these obstacles is critical to your mental well-being at work. I've found there are three big obstacles that commonly trip us up during the day:

OBSTACLE #1: GETTING EMOTIONALLY HIJACKED

You know that feeling. There's tension in your muscles. You're starting to feel irritable, blaming other people for missed deadlines or mistakes, and you're making impulsive decisions or rash comments—in short, you're falling "below the line" big time. And if you start to feel sadness, stress, frustration, anger, or even rage building up inside, it's a sign your emotions have hijacked your brain into a state that is both unproductive and unhealthy. You risk saying something or doing something that could be hurtful to other people and your position both short and long term.

OBSTACLE # 2: FEELING UNMOTIVATED

You feel exhausted and ready to give up on your day or a project. You feel sluggish, tired, or bored. You may procrastinate or avoid working on projects you need to get done or only answer the most urgent emails. You start to check out on what is happening around you. There's a deadness and numbness inside of you, and you can feel your heart rate start to slow down. Your emails are piling up unanswered, your project timelines are falling further and further behind, and it all begins to feel hopeless and worthless. At its worst, feeling unmotivated makes you not even want to get out of bed in the morning. *Please note, if this feeling goes on for several weeks or longer, consider speaking to your Employee Assistance Program (EAP) or a professional counselor.*

OBSTACLE #3: DIFFICULT INTERACTIONS

Why is it that some days all it takes is a simple question or remark from someone at work for you to feel threatened or get defensive? I'm very fortunate that I have an amazing manager. However, in a recent touch-base meeting, my manager reminded me of all I had on my plate for the coming week. We had discussed this list of projects in a previous discussion, and I started to feel myself get frustrated and overwhelmed at this reminder. I had to check in with myself and realize that I was interpreting her reminder as being a micromanager. And I've always bristled at being micromanaged. Her innocent comments triggered me that day, and since that is an unusual reaction, I paused to reflect that evening. It turns out that I had a very challenging client call a couple hours before, and I never took time to check in after, address and regulate my emotional responses, and be Brain On! I was still operating in emotional hijack mode when I met with my manager and carried that emotional baggage with me to my next meeting. It's like driving with a dirty windshield. You just can't think and interpret things clearly. That is why these frequent check-ins with yourself to make sure you remain Brain On! are so critical.

Notice how the first two obstacles are responses to negative internal emotions and feelings, while the third is a negative response to external stimuli. Going back to Chapter 2 and the daily obstacle course, this is what we called the internal and external obstacles. All these obstacles need to be overcome by staying Brain On! through regulating and steadying our emotional reactions. Our task throughout the day is to manage the inner obstacles first, as those impact how we handle our external obstacles. What is going on inside of you influences your perception and reaction to the work environment around you, which influences the choices you make, the actions you take, and what you achieve each day. Going back to the situation with my manager: I was brain off in that discussion when we were just talking about my project list. Imagine if I came into that meeting while being brain off, and she was giving me a performance review, or we were discussing an issue or mistake? I wouldn't have taken any of that news constructively. I could have easily spiraled into "I hate my job, and I don't feel appreciated," and our relationship would have deteriorated quickly.

Mental Fitness Exercises to Leap Over the Obstacles

Ready to build some mental strength to overcome your daily obstacle course? Here are some easy practices that take just a few moments out of your day. Many of them you can do at your desk or even in a meeting.

EXERCISES FOR EMOTIONAL HIJACKING

When negative emotions like anger, sadness, or fear start bubbling up, take a moment to do an emotional check-in using these exercises:

Exercise #1: What am I feeling?

Be specific with your emotional state, or "name it to tame it." Noted author and psychiatrist Dr. Daniel Siegel coined this phrase as a simple tool that can work to regulate your emotions. We typically describe our emotions in six broad categories—anger, contempt, disgust, fear, happiness, sadness, and surprise. When you use more specific terms, it helps you put more distance and perspective around your feelings. Am I sad versus disappointed? Do I feel anger, or is it really frustration? Am I tired or just bored? Specifically identifying your emotion correctly allows your brain to process it more effectively and efficiently.

Exercise #2: What am I thinking?

Dr. Darren Weissman, author of *Awakening the Secret Code of Your Mind*,[22] suggests asking yourself: Would I ever choose to feel (insert the unpleasant emotion you are feeling)? The answer is probably NO! He calls this uncomfortable feeling a "gift in strange wrapping paper." It's helping you recognize you've been emotionally hijacked and your thinking brain is offline.

Exercise #3: What are the stories I'm telling myself right now?

Are you repeating in your head negative stories that are drummed up from past slights or rejections? When things aren't clear or certain, our brain likes to fill in the blanks to close the loop and add closure to the situation. Your manager or colleague might look at you with a raised brow, and the story you immediately tell yourself is that they are mad at you or you did something wrong. Or you receive an abbreviated email from a client saying, "Call me when you get a chance," and you assume it's an issue or problem. You receive a meeting request during a time you are overwhelmed, and you immediately say this will be a waste of time and become instantly frustrated and agitated. The exercise here is to examine the storyline and replace it with a better story. Byron Katie, best-selling author and creator of The Work, which is a process to apply questions to any problems, suggests asking yourself: Is this true? Can you absolutely know it's true (100 percent sure)? How do you react? What happens when you believe those thoughts or the story you are telling yourself? Who would you be without that thought?

EXERCISES WHEN FEELING UNMOTIVATED

Breathwork and meditation have so many emotional and health benefits. These mental fitness exercises can be practiced during those moments at work when you need to bring your energy back and your brain online. Breathwork has been proven to help bring greater focus to a task and to enhance creativity and problem-solving. Simply focusing on your breath activates your parasympathetic nervous system to "turn on" your thinking brain and put the brakes on your emotional brain from continuing to take charge. A short meditation practice can refresh your attention at work.

Exercise #1: Breathe in calm.

As you inhale and exhale through your nose, say these words to yourself, "Breathe in calm, breathe out peace." You are training your brain to pay attention to the words, while creating a sense of peace by using these types of words. This helps divert your focus away from the event that caused the emotional hijacking and prevents you from continuing to downward spiral by re-playing it in your head over and over. I repeat this practice ten to fifteen times every time I find myself emotionally reactive and in brain-off mode. Sometimes I use the word "joy" instead of "peace." Whatever creates a relaxed and slightly happy mood for you. Once you've got this exercise down, try the advanced version by extending your out breath for a couple seconds longer than your in breath as your repeat these words. This is a powerful and easy way to calm your nervous system and bring your thinking brain back online.

Exercise #2: Three deep breaths.

On the first breath, try to let go of any thoughts racing in your mind. On the second breath, relax your body to melt the tension away, and on the third breath, bring to mind someone or something (like your pet) that you care for that makes you smile and silently wish them well.

Exercise #3: Square breathing.

People love this practice because it is so simple but has amazing benefits. It heightens performance and concentration while reducing stress. Everyone from athletes to police officers use this four-step, four-count practice:

1. Inhale air through your nose for a count of four.
2. Hold and keep the air in your lungs for a count of four.
3. Expel the air through the nose for a count of four.
4. Hold and keep your lungs empty for a count of four.

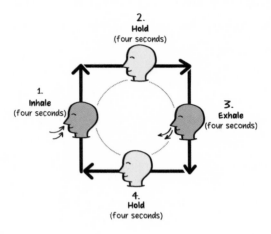

2.
Hold
(four seconds)

1.
Inhale
(four seconds)

3.
Exhale
(four seconds)

4.
Hold
(four seconds)

Exercise #4: Body scan.

This practice can be done at your desk, sitting on a park bench, or waiting for your plane to take off. A seated meditation can help you recharge before you feel your head fall to your desk in utter depletion and exhaustion. These guided steps come from the book *Finding the Space to Lead: A Practical Guide to Mindful Leadership* by Janice Marturano.[23]

Begin by bringing your attention to the sensations of your breath.

When you're ready, direct your attention to the soles of your feet, opening your mind to whatever sensations are there to be noticed.

Perhaps you are noticing the pressure on the soles of your feet as the weight of your legs rest on them. Perhaps the soles of your feet feel warm or cool.

Just notice. No need to judge or engage in discursive thinking. If your mind is pulled away or wanders, redirect your attention, firmly and gently.

Move your attention next to the tops of your feet, ankles, lower legs, knees, and so forth.

Gradually scan through your body, noticing sensations, noticing discomfort, and noticing areas of your body where you detect an absence of sensations. No need to search for sensations; just keep scanning through your body, taking your time and being open to what is here.

EXERCISES FOR DIFFICULT INTERACTIONS

The practices I just presented were meant to help you regulate your emotions to manage the inner game. But your workday is all about those human and external interactions, whether it's a client, co-worker, manager, or someone else in your work sphere. Think about some of the external obstacles you've had lately that threw your thinking brain off. Did you receive an email request while already overwhelmed and fall into frustration? Did you hear of someone else getting the project you wanted or a promotion and fall into a state of rejection or victim mode? Were you depressed after being left out of an important meeting that effects your job responsibility? Sometimes all it takes is one of your co-workers having a really bad day, and they respond to you in a harsh tone or raised voice. Those negative emotions are contagious and can impact your day, even though it's not about you.

Exercise #1: Pause.

The first step to take when we realize we're operating "below the line" in these situations is to stop and be willing to pause. I often remind myself of what philosopher Viktor Frankl said, "Between the stimulus and the response, there is a space. And in that space is our power and our freedom." I once heard *Emotional Intelligence* author Daniel Goleman share in a training that the definition of maturity is the length of that pause before a reaction. I believe emotional maturity is a lifelong journey, and it's the journey with the most rewards.

Exercise #2: RAIN.

When I find myself reacting negatively to reactions from a manager, team member, or client, one of the most powerful practices I turn to is Tara Brach's RAIN practice. She is a renowned meditation teacher, psychologist, and author of several books, including *Radical Compassion: Learning to Love Yourself and Your World with the Practice of RAIN*.[24] The acronym stands for:

> *Recognize what is happening.*
> *Allow and accept the experience to be there, just as it is.*
> *Investigate with interest and care.*
> *Nurture with self-compassion.*

Recognize what is happening is all about naming the emotion you are feeling as accurately as possible, as I mentioned earlier in this chapter.

Allow the experience to be there, and accept it —this is a huge step that many of us bypass. Acceptance of the situation is critical; otherwise you will continue to suffer over your reaction. The phrase "what you resist, persists" rings true here. If you want to free yourself of the emotional hangover of a negative reaction, allow the acceptance to flow.

Investigate is understanding where the pain about the situation is coming from. Be a little like a private detective and try to solve where those negative emotions, thoughts, or feelings are coming from.

Nurture with compassion, both toward yourself and others. To do this, I might do one of those quick breathing exercises, journal, or go for a walk.

Honestly, I find myself practicing RAIN daily because of all the emotional obstacles at work. I find that I notice my emotions when I catch myself verbalizing them.

"I'm so frustrated."

"Oh, I'm disappointed in that decision."

"This email makes me so mad."

Or I notice and pay more attention to the emotions I'm feeling when I get a twinge in my neck, feel a knot in my shoulders, or get an upset stomach or headache from stress. I've trained my brain to notice and pay attention to these cues that indicate I've been emotionally hijacked and my thinking brain is now offline.

The hardest part of the RAIN practice for me is allowing and accepting. I'm one that likes to stuff my emotions down or put on a happy face. I've learned over the years that it has significant health as well as productivity consequences for me. Jeremy

Hunter, founding director of the Executive Mind Leadership Institute, said something that really helped me realize the importance of this concept. "Acceptance is the key to reducing suffering, anguish, anger, and rumination," he said. When I felt I was under the microscope for my performance, I just breathed and allowed my feelings of frustration to be there. I did not just ignore them. I accepted the situation, especially if a mistake was made. No sense reliving it in my mind because that just prolongs my suffering.

Investigate is my favorite part of RAIN. I relish playing the private investigator with compassionate curiosity and trying to discover what is going on and why I'm feeling this way. When I do this, I learn how irrational some of my thinking is on a very innocent exchange with a co-worker. Or how I was adding and believing my own storyline I made up about the situation. This would explain why I felt my jaw or fist clenched an hour later. Or why I would get a headache or feel exhausted at other times. This insight has been invaluable in terms of building a healthier relationship with my brain and body, as well as my manager, team, and clients. A true win-win.

Nurture involves self-kindness, which many people find difficult to give. That includes me. I can be my own worst enemy! When I fall into negative self-talk, I ask myself: would I say those things to my child, friend, or loved one? Would you treat them that way if they made the same mistake you did? No! You'd say, "It's okay." And then you'd shower them with kindness and compassion. Showing compassion for ourselves and others is the humanness that connects us all. Some nurturing phrases I use that connect us to others include, "I like to be happy and so does this person." "I want to be healthy and so does this person." "I cry sometimes and so does this person." "I feel pain sometimes and so does this person." "I'm trying my best and so is this person."

Final Exercise: Gratitude for your brain.

The final brain exercise you can incorporate each day, and the one that can keep you energized for the next day, is to be grateful for how your brain performed that day. There is no better way to transition from the workday or even get a good night's sleep than with a big dose of gratitude.

If your day didn't go as you hoped, consider this quote from Tom Rath's book, *Life's Great Question*, "When you're struggling at work or have a bad day, try reconstructing your most recent day (or week) and looking for tasks you may be able to fine-tune in terms of where you invest time and energy. Consider how the use of each hour is of additional benefit to the people you serve. We have to do a better job of connecting practical daily actions with purpose."

In positive psychology research, gratitude is strongly and consistently associated with greater happiness. Gratitude helps people feel more positive emotions, relish good experiences, improve their health, deal with adversity, and build strong relationships. And it's easy. Psychologist Martin Seligman, known as the "father of positive psychology," developed this quick, but meaningful practice:

Each night before you go to sleep:

1. Think of three good things that happened today.
2. Write them down.
3. Reflect on why they happened (and how they made you feel).[25]

This exercise took a while for me to consistently practice and make a habit. But it was worth it. It has changed my life for the better, and on top of that, I can flip back and look at so many wonderful moments. This gratitude practice elicits positive emotions and I feel Brain On! Scott Shute, author of *The Full Body Yes: Change Your Work and Your World from the Inside Out*, says that gratitude is a superpower.[26] I couldn't agree more.

CHAPTER 8
ON-DEMAND BRAIN BOOSTERS

"I'm Brain On! But still dragging."

It's a fresh morning at work. You've cleared your calendar to dig into a new project and removed all distractions like email and text notifications. You're feeling calm and rational, and not feeling at all emotionally hijacked. Brain On? Check. But you still are having trouble mustering up the energy to get started. For some reason you're feeling blah, and all you want to do is put your head down for a nap even though your day is barely started. Or you just can't get past that midday slump even with your third cup of coffee. What's up with that?

Remember, there are two steps to ensure you have an energizing day at work. The first is checking that you are Brain On! and that your thinking brain is keeping you emotionally regulated and thinking clearly. These are all the things we covered in Chapter 7, especially assessing throughout your workday if you are operating above the line (open, curious, listening, trusting). The second step is to get into the Energizer mode by keeping your brain's battery powered up. Your goal is to maintain your brain's energy throughout the day, so by the end, you'll feel as energized as you started.

I do believe, and have witnessed, that people can improve their mental well-being at work by boosting their brain's energy level. If you let your brain get run down each day, you begin a downward spiral in mood that can ruin your evening or even hang over you for days. When you leave work with as much or even more energy as you started with that morning, it creates an upward spiral of positivity that energizes you in all parts of your life, including with friends and family members.

Like your body, your brain has its own set of daily essentials that it needs to stay strong and energized. We've already covered the cognitive essentials your brain needs, such as setting strengths-based goals to keep your brain focused. Mental fitness exercises, such as breathing, meditation, and the RAIN practice, increase your self-awareness and keep your thinking brain on. Brain boosters are the final daily essentials—these are energy management techniques that can recharge your brain power and provide sparks of energy throughout your day.

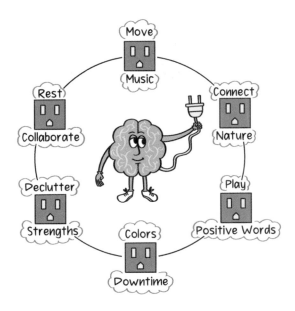

Brain Booster #1

Rest for success

The days of being a superhero by surviving on four hours of sleep are over. So are the days of sitting in front of our computer screens for ten hours straight and not giving our eyes and brains some relief. Our brain needs rest and recovery time. Poor sleep has been linked to higher rates of blood pressure, diabetes, obesity, anxiety, depression, and reduced immune function. Being rest-starved makes you cranky and distracted, forgetful and easily short-circuited, and brain off. Getting a good night's sleep is critical to brain function as well as emotional regulation. Even naps as short as twenty minutes can give your brain an energy boost.

Brain Booster #2

Move frequently

Moving your body improves your mood, energy, and productivity. Sitting for more than thirty minutes changes how your body is functioning. Getting up to move around every thirty minutes or so is proven to help your thinking, creativity, and cognitive abilities. If you can't get up every thirty minutes, try aiming for a five-minute stand, stroll, or stretch every hour. At minimum, try to work at a sit-stand desk, or aim for standing at least fifteen minutes an hour while on a call.

Brain Booster #3

Connect with others

Connecting with other people is one of the mental nutrients in the The Healthy Mind Platter™ created by Dr. David Rock, executive director of the NeuroLeadership Institute, and Dr. Daniel Siegel ("name it to tame it"), executive director of the Mindsight Institute and clinical professor at the UCLA School of Medicine.[27] Drs. Rock and Siegel explain that when you make connections with other people, it richly activates and improves the brain's circuitry. Make time for short, but meaningful connections during the day. Find a colleague at work you enjoy collaborating with and spend a few moments with them. Or call your partner or a friend and take a few minutes to catch up.

Brain Booster #4

Play more

Incorporating play into your workday is not a trivial pursuit. Being spontaneous and creative forges new connections in the brain, and can combat fatigue, stress, and burnout. The easiest way to incorporate play into your workday is to simply laugh. Laughter increases your brain's release of endorphins and dopamine that stimulate circulation and aid muscle relaxation. Daniel Pink, the award-winning *New York Times* bestselling author, wrote in his book *A Whole New Mind*, "It's time to rescue humor from its status as mere entertainment and recognize it for what it is—a sophisticated and peculiarly human form of intelligence that can't be replicated by computers and that is becoming increasingly valuable in a high-concept, high-touch world."[28]

Sharing humorous stories with your colleagues or reminiscing about a fun event you both attended can add some much-needed humor and stress reduction to your day. I begin many of my presentations with a humorous comment or illustration to help relax my audience and open up their creative thinking on a new topic. Play can also just refer to introducing something novel, just to shake off the cobwebs. The brain gets energy from seeing new, novel things. Pull out the daily crossword puzzle, sudoku, quick online game, or brain teaser to spark a little energy and get you going. Just make sure to avoid those addictive games where five minutes turns into fifty minutes.

Brain Booster #5

Schedule downtime

Breaks were one of the six strategies for an energizing day that I outlined in Chapter 6. I'm reinforcing the benefits of taking a time out again in this list because they are critical in improving your energy and mental focus at any point when you need a brain boost. Here's the easiest time out you can give yourself, and one that is good for both your body and brain. Once an hour, get up and refill your water bottle or brew a cup of herbal tea.

Brain Booster #6

Collaborate for motivation

We explored the importance of aligning your strengths to your work each day in Chapter 5 to stay in the Energizer mode. Sometimes finding the motivation to move forward with your strengths-based projects can get a boost by collaborating with a colleague. When I'm jotting down new ideas or focused on creating new frameworks, I'm aligned to my futurist, ideation, maximizer strengths. But when I sit down and try to write out all the details, I immediately lose motivation and energy. It becomes a tedious, dreadful chore. Why? Well at the bottom of my strengths list is Communication and Context. It's like swimming upstream in a hurricane. I found if I can partner with someone good at this, like my collaborative writer Melinda Cross, I'm much more energized and happier.

Brain Booster #7

Music to improve your mood

Music has been proven to improve your productivity, cognitive performance, and mood. Just ask any music therapist. Listening to music can help you manage anxiety and increase motivation. The trick is to start out with slower-paced music when you have low energy. Gradually increase the tempo of the songs and choose music with little to no lyrics that can be distractions. When I was writing this book and facing pages and pages of edits and rewrites, I found video game music stimulating.

Brain Booster #8

Be in nature

Research has shown that working in and around nature can help people be more focused and productive. In fact, biophilia (incorporating nature into the workplace) has become a focus for improving productivity as well as mood. If possible, take a short walk outside during the day and observe the trees, flowers, grass, or sun around you. At minimum, try to spend time near a window with a pleasant view of nature while working or having a meeting. Or even have a plant on your desk or have beautiful landscapes as your screen saver on your computer.

Choose positive words

Change your words and you can change your energy. Using the right words can raise your energy levels and motivation. Try and catch yourself from using negative self-talk or making self-deprecating remarks. Post positive and inspirational quotes on your desktop or office walls. Incorporate positive adjectives and responses in your conversation, even words as simple as "great, terrific, I appreciate that." On those days you are feeling particularly low energy, those are the days to steer clear of negative news and online gossip and strategically surround yourself with friends and colleagues that have a positive view on things so you can draw from their positive energy to fuel yours.

Brain Booster #10

Add color

I've always loved color on the walls in my home and company office. When I found out that studies showed color increases productivity and creativity, it made sense. Too much gray, beige, and white in offices can feel sterile or depressing, especially in geographic areas that don't see much sun in the winter. There are color psychologists who help companies choose the right hues for their offices to create a specific mood, such as orange for energy, yellow for positivity, green for harmony, and blue for relaxation. And you can opt for an easy brain boost by adding color to your workstation. Small artwork, colored stones in a vase (with a plant), or even a colored frame add a boost for your brain every time you glance at it.

Brain Booster #11

Clear the clutter

You've probably heard the phrase "cluttered desk, cluttered mind." Even if you're a person who isn't bothered by stacks of files on your desk, research has shown that our brains do like order. Seeing visual disorganization can hinder our ability to focus. Scientists at the Princeton University Neuroscience Institute discovered that when people cleared the clutter from their offices, they could better process information which increased productivity.

Schedule Your Daily Boosts

These techniques contribute to the energy management of my brain every day. I have days when I forget to give my brain the self-care and energy boosts it needs because I'm balancing a jam-packed work schedule while playing air traffic controller for my family's needs. That's when the trouble starts—I get edgy with co-workers, short with my husband and children, and even the dog wants to steer clear of me.

> BRAIN CHECK: Now, let's put it all together. Take a few minutes to jot down how you can begin to incorporate these brain boosters into your day:
>
> - Rest
> - Movement
> - Connection
> - Play
> - Downtime
> - Strengths

- Music
- Nature
- Words

- Colors
- Decluttering

My Brain Booster Strategies

_____

_____

_____

There's no specific recipe for an energized mind, as each person is different, and it depends on our workday and the obstacles we encounter that day. The point is it's not only critical to check in often to make sure you are Brain On!, but that you have a fully charged battery at various points throughout the day. And if you don't, and you feel depleted or your energy dipping, building in the habit to use one of these brain boosters to recharge your batteries. That is the only way to end your day better than you started and be in Energizer mode when the day is done.

A fun use of this idea is to reflect each day on when your energy dipped and what really brought you back to life. For me, I know if I start out the day with low energy, it means I didn't sleep well, and the only antidote is scheduling a twenty-minute power nap or meditation. Around 2 p.m. When I'm just dragging, I know to get up, stretch, and step outside in nature. Or on rainy days, get up and play my favorite pick-me-up song. The point here is there are many combinations that can work well and over time you will be able to train your brain to use the brain boosters that work well for you and build in these important habits into your daily routine.

PART TWO HIGHLIGHT REEL

We've covered a lot of mental fitness exercises to stay Brain On! and have an Energizer day. Here is a summary of highlights you can use for a quick refresher in the morning, during lunch, or on your afternoon break:

- The relationship you have with your brain is a top priority. How we regulate our brain's responses and coach it into a healthy condition is what ensures we have a positive and fulfilling day.

- There are two key ingredients to managing your brain for an Energizer day. The first is setting, prioritizing, and taking action on your strengths-based goals. The second is managing the energy of your brain.

- *How* you achieve your goals is equally as important as *what* you achieve. The key to your well-being is to emotionally regulate your brain to avoid stress and burnout on the way to achieving your goals.

- Primary mental fitness goals: Stay Brain On! and achieve and stay in Energizer mode so you have the brain power and motivation to achieve your strengths-based goals in the workplace.

- Knowing your strengths-based goals keeps you motivated. Focusing on aligning our strengths with our goals is something we aren't taught and don't take time to do.

- Accept that every day is going to have some obstacles. Knowing and accepting this fact goes a long way in not beating yourself up when your brain starts to go offline, and you feel its energy depleting

- The primary function of your thinking brain at work is to keep you operating at optimal performance. When your emotional brain goes into autopilot and overrides your thinking brain, it's difficult, if not impossible, to perform critical tasks at work.

- Stay aware of the triggers. Most people have three broad signals that their brain is going offline, and it's time to get it back on track with some simple practices: 1) Getting emotionally hijacked, 2) Feeling unmotivated, 3) Difficult interactions with manager, team, or clients.

- Prioritizing self-care with Brain Boosters. Actively planning your day to include enough rest, nature, music, play, connection, and more will restore your brain's energy when you are feeling it drop or the brain drain.

CONGRATULATIONS! If you've read this far, you've successfully learned what it means to be Brain On! at work and have strategies and tactics to win your workday and keep those pesky obstacles from hijacking you and sapping your energy. As I mentioned at the start of the book, you may not need to go on to Part Three if you aren't a leader, HR team member, or in charge of organizational initiatives. But if you are in one of those roles, or curious how the Brain On! approach applies to managing teams, people, and an organization, please read on!

PART THREE
BRAIN ON! ORGANIZATIONAL PLAYBOOK

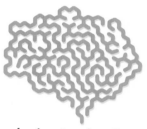

You've now learned what it takes for an individual to keep themselves Brain On! through emotional regulation and staying energized. Chances are, either now or at some point in your career, you will be leading, managing, or have other direct influence on your colleagues in a smaller team, a larger group, or maybe an entire organization.

How you show up emotionally as a leader, an HR professional, or an executive responsible for setting the cultural tone of the organization can be more impactful to employees than pay, promotions, or perks. There is the real possibility that the wrong words or actions during the workday could be perceived as a threat and trigger an employee's alarm system instead of keeping them Brain On! The small conversations and interactions you have during the day can make or break productivity, creativity, and happiness at work for yourself and others.

We've learned that our brain's natural default mode is brain off. At the end of the day, people running organizations and setting their policies need to be aware that it is their responsibility to keep people in a positive energy state and create workdays that are regenerative. Marcus Buckingham, business consultant and author of *StandOut* and *Nine Lies About Work*, often reminds his audiences that people quit managers, not jobs. In the new Brain On! way of managing and leading people, your task differs somewhat depending on your role:

- A leader leads other brains.
- An HR team leads the collective brain.
- An organization transforms the collective brain.

This Organization Playbook is written for all these positions of leadership. My goal with this section is to reinforce that your emotions are contagious, and the actions you take and words you choose are never neutral. You can either help remove barriers and obstacles in people's workdays or create more of them. You are responsible for keeping them Brain On! by eliminating any work triggers and helping to avoid hijacking their emotions. This will ultimately determine if they have an energizing day instead of feeling burned out, disengaged, or disconnected.

Think of the individual employee's experience. You've learned that they bring their own internal barriers and obstacles to the workday. But it is their leaders, HR team and its policies, and the organizational culture that ultimately determine the Brain On! and Energizer workday.

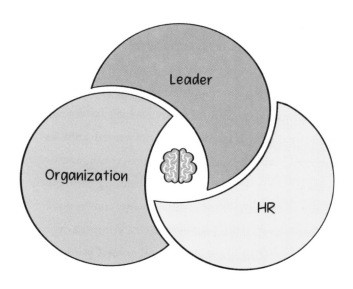

This visual illuminates how myriad interactions and communications from throughout the organization can pop up for individual employees and trigger new emotions and thoughts throughout the day. Some they were planning for, and some they weren't. Most will hopefully trigger their brain's reward system in a positive way and keep their thinking brain on. Others may create obstacles that shut an employee's brain down and halt their productivity. As a leader, are you consciously aware of how your message, your body language, and your interactions create a threat or reward? Do these interactions strengthen or deteriorate your relationship with the employee in that moment? These are critical questions for you to keep in mind to answer throughout your workday as they impact the employee experience in either positive or negative ways. A co-worker once said something long ago that continues to ring true for me as a parent. You are only as happy as your unhappiest child. This also applies to your organization. It is only as productive, innovative, and successful as your unhappiest or most unmotivated employee or team member.

This lesson is especially important to keep in mind during your organization's most demanding season, which is typically the end of the fiscal year. This is when your entire organization as a collective brain could be at its most fragile, stressed-out, and unhappiest. Employees feel that additional pressure running through the organization through all the potentially negative and "brain-off" interactions coming from managers and leaders. For most organizations, this period is October through December, or Q4 of the calendar year. (I recognize that some organizations are on a July 1 or October 1 fiscal year, or benefit plan year, so the months leading up to those dates are the brain-off period).

For employees, this end-of-the-year period is filled with even more personal and work-related obstacles that keep mounting as the days tick by toward the year-end finish line.

Additional obstacles for leaders and the HR team to be aware of during this time include:

- Organizational budgets due.
- Pay increases and year-end bonuses to be determined.
- Client holiday entertaining and holiday team parties to plan.

- Not enough resources during busy season.
- Internal requests from auditors and compliance trying to wrap up year-end.
- Pressure to make your year-end revenue goals.
- Annual enrollment with town halls and benefits meetings need to be offered.
- Goals for the next year need to be developed.

Additional obstacles for individual employees include:

- Not enough resources to handle Q4 business needs.
- Facing stressful family holidays.
- Worry about children's finals and semester ending for working parents.
- Creating goals for the new year.
- Day care issues with holiday breaks.
- Juggling doctor appointments and medical procedures since most deductibles have been satisfied by Q4.
- Financial stress increases as the holiday shopping season starts.
- Increased demands on time with holiday parties and client celebrations.
- Trying to squeeze in remaining vacation amidst tight year-end deadlines.
- Pressure to select annual benefits.
- News about end-of-year bonuses and next year's pay raise.

Just reading this you might notice a slight increase in your stress level or tension in your body as your brain recalls these activities or time frame. This is the point, and the great opportunity for leaders to change how the people in your organization react and communicate during those busy or challenging times. This Organizational Playbook will help you better understand and improve your mental strength as well as individuals in your organization. Flipping the script with each of these scenarios using the Brain On! approach is critical if you want to create a better way to work, thrive, and be successful in your goals.

In the following chapters of the Brain On! Organizational Playbook, I'm going to outline how a leader, HR team member, and overall culture of an organization all contribute to developing a mentally strong organization—one that is even more resilient and productive during the busiest time of year. My belief and what I've experienced throughout my career is that a mentally strong organization doesn't happen unless each of the individuals in leadership roles first ensures they are operating Brain On!—checking to make sure their own oxygen mask is on, and they are energized themselves. After all, leaders are people, too, with their own set of emotions to manage each day. Mental well-being starts at the top. And as the great leadership expert Peter Drucker first proposed in his book *Managing Oneself,* **you cannot manage others until you manage yourself.** So that is where we begin. Focusing on you as a leader.

CHAPTER 9

THE INNER GAME OF BEING A BRAIN ON! LEADER

"How do I keep other brains in Energizer mode?"

There are a lot of terrific books on leadership and management, and you probably have many on your shelf as they can give you tremendously effective strategies and techniques on how to manage business strategy, operations, financial skills, and other work skills. What I've found is that having great business acumen and career achievements doesn't necessarily give you the Brain On! people skills necessary to keep your team high functioning and mentally strong. This is the difference between the old definition of a business leaders and the new, human-centered, Brain On! leader. Some call these critically necessary and differentiating qualities "soft skills," but that term makes it sound less important than the work- and job-specific skills. I like to use the term human skills or interpersonal skills as these are equally important, if not more so, to becoming a great leader than any other knowledge or set of business skills in today's world. Think of your leadership role first as that of being a team captain. You need to be the best at using these mental fitness skills and then model them to train and support your individual employees in how to be Brain On! and energized throughout the day on the playing field. People look to you, their team captain, for inspiration and guidance, and to exemplify what successful attitudes and behaviors look like while at work. Most importantly, when they are low energy and feeling unmotivated or not performing at their best, employees look to you for inspiration and to help them stay Brain On! and get back to Energizer mode as well. This chapter is designed to "train the trainer"—you!

A leader's main task throughout the day is to consciously and consistently check in to see if they are Brain On! before making decisions, performing tasks, and in every interaction with another person. Do you feel distracted, tired, frustrated, or even angry? Feelings that indicate you are coming from a place of brain off? Could these negative or toxic emotions be having a detrimental impact on your team or relationships with your colleagues? If so, you need to use the same strategies and techniques we covered in Part Two (like pausing before proceeding) to regulate yourself emotionally and manage your inner game to create a positive and visible energy that will engage and motivate employees in that interaction or communication.

The difference between being an individual brain in the workplace and being a leader is that you need to check in with yourself many more times during the day because your emotions can ripple far and wide. You likely have several or even a dozen more daily people interactions as you manage up, down, and across the organization and in all communication formats—virtually, digitally, and in person. No one expects you to be perfect as a person. You're going to get distracted, upset, and stressed just like anyone else. But here's the rub—your negative or fear-based emotion can be contagious and trigger employees into a brain-off mode at any time, resulting in lower energy and engagement, a deterioration of your relationships, and less productive conversations and a less productive working environment for everyone.

Here is what I consider the leader's training circuit—the additional core building blocks and mental fitness exercises necessary to be a Brain On! and energizing leader.

The Leader's Brain On! Training Circuit

As we discussed, leaders are people too and therefore should focus on their own mental well-being first by practicing and mastering the skills we discussed in the Individual Playbook just like everyone else. But to truly be an effective Brain On! leader there is an additional leadership training circuit that you can use throughout your day to strengthen specific leadership mental muscles necessary and help you master your inner game as team captain. It's like weightlifting. You do exercises to strengthen your core, which we did in Part One, the Individual Playbook. And then you do isolation exercises to develop, define, and strengthen specific muscles like your arms, legs, back. That is what we are doing with the leadership training circuit. Isolating the key mental muscles that will make you a Brain On! and Energizer leader.

Here is what I consider the leader's training circuit. There are six stations or exercises that leaders need to also focus on and master. These go beyond and much deeper than the skills highlighted in many of the leadership books you read. These exercises are specifically meant to strengthen your greatest asset as a leader: your brain. The six check-in stations can be easily remembered through this mnemonic: C-A-P-T-A-I-N. These exercises will take you from a good "business" leader with some human skills to a great human leader with amazing business skills. These will take you from a person people look to for direction and are required to follow to a leader that people look to for inspiration and want to follow.

BE A BRAIN ON! TEAM C-A-P-T-A-I-N

C – Check-in with yourself frequently to see if you are Brain On! or brain off.

A – Align with your strengths, in your job tasks as well as your goals.

P – Pause purposefully before any interaction (verbal or virtual) to ensure you're Brain On!

T – Talk less; listen more. Lead with curiosity and compassion in all conversations.

A – Acknowledge and recognize each team member's small and large contributions often.

I – Initiate growth to ensure you and your team are constantly learning new things and growing.

N – Navigate the difficult conversations. Stay present, Brain On!, and speak from a place of compassion.

Almost all great leadership books ask you to reflect about your behavior and performance. But they are usually externally focused, high-level, and business related. The Brain On! approach addresses the gap between external and internal and emotional performance by asking the right questions to uncover how we are leading as human beings. These Brain On! check-ins are strategically structured to ask the key questions of yourself applied to your emotional regulation and contagion during the workday. Basic mental hygiene questions will lead to stronger mental well-being and a Brain On! and energizing day for both you and those around you.

A book by leadership consultant John Maxwell, *Good Leaders Ask Great Questions,* emphasizes the need to get very skilled at the art of asking questions. What the leadership circuit accomplishes is building a great daily habit of asking and answering key leadership questions that are focused on specifically transforming and rewiring your brain, your day, and your work. Then modeling that and training others to do the same.

Check-in Station #1

Am I aware of my present, real-time thoughts and emotions?

The answer is probably no for most of us and almost all the time.

The concept of individual check-ins was discussed in Part Two, and they become your foundation in becoming a great Brain On! Leader. As a leader, you are moving so fast and handling so many things that you may be operating brain off more than you realize. You're not as focused, clear, and effective as you can be. If you respond too quickly to things you don't like, you risk saying or doing things that won't be particularly kind, wise, or useful to your team.

After checking in with yourself, part two of this exercise to build strong mental muscles as a leader is to take a pause. Practice pausing before reacting or responding, and witness how that makes you a more "level-headed" person and leader—that is the exercise to practice and master at this circuit station. And there are numerous times during the day you can do a "rep" or two. Pause before sending that email, entering that meeting, answering a work text, or before any interaction with an employee, team member, or client. Every time you pause before speaking or acting too quickly, you are doing one repetition in your training, and these reps can easily add up to twenty or thirty times a day. The length of your pause determines how strong you are and defines your leadership maturity.

Think of how a team captain will call a timeout—that's a purposeful pause in the action and can be the key to winning a game. Team captains also call a timeout if they think the team players are brain off and need to regroup to get back online, work better together, and win their workday.

Am I effectively using my strengths in all situations and moving toward my own strengths-based goals?

A leader faces a very demanding and busy workday often dictated by their calendar. This requires the utmost efficiency and effectiveness to achieve results. Operating Brain On! is step one, so everything comes from a place of clarity and focus and is intentional. The second exercise is making sure your goals, even daily goals, align with your strengths, gifts, and talents. To do so often means delegating to others or finding a partner to handle those responsibilities that don't play into your strengths. For example, if you need to create a team presentation or an executive communication and inspirational writing is not one of your strengths, this needs to be delegated to someone with that creative talent. If your strength is achieving results but not envisioning the necessary future enhancements or changes, you'll need to find a strategic partner that is innovative to help co-create that vision you desire to execute and achieve. It's not that you can't do all the necessary parts of your job. It's just we need to realize we aren't wired to be great at everything. Certain things will feel like you are swimming upstream in a tidal wave, leaving you exhausted or demotivated.

Leading through others is a sign of great leadership, especially when you align strategically with other's strengths to balance out yours. This is why it's just as important to know your strengths as it is to understand what you are not wired for as well. Homing in on what lights you up and ensuring those skills are being fully utilized every day and for most of that day will make you more successful as a leader, mentally stronger, and more energized. It will inspire others to do the same.

Check-in Station #3

Am I tuned into the thoughts and feelings of others?

This exercise might seem easy and one you might think you don't need to practice or incorporate into your daily exercise routine. However, if you remember your brain is constantly scanning for threats, mind wandering up to 50 percent of the time and primarily focusing on you, your experience, and your safety, chances are you aren't really listening to or reading all the words or empathizing with all the feelings being communicated by another. Deep listening is all about being curious. That is the mental muscle you are building in this exercise. As you aim to learn more, by staying present, focused on the other, and curious, that is one "rep." In all conversations, you are like a private investigator trying to uncover the key messages and sentiments that will build a stronger connection and better results with each conversation or exchange. Do you use that as your goal in your conversations? Instead of dictating or being center stage, do you aim to have a true dialogue? The most effective three words a leader can use to show they are deeply listening is, "Tell me more."

I have seen amazing results and relationships built when a leader uses this technique in various ways during conversations to dig deep and get at the root issue or main point of the dialogue instead of jumping in too quickly and trying to address or fix only the surface level issue. Ask your team member to share examples of what is working or not working for them or to clarify what they are describing. As a deep listener, you're trying to collect enough data by asking enough questions so that you see the issue or request clearly and respond appropriately from a position of intelligence and empathy to continue to have a productive and effective conversation (versus responding from your own perception, stories, and assumptions and having an unproductive conversation). Being a good listener also means suspending judgment during the conversation. Or wanting to tell them how to fix things before you even know the real issue.

The exercise becomes: Can you have a conversation without saying what you think is right or use examples without you in them? I'm sure you can think of a time you were talking to another person about something you were experiencing or a challenge you were facing, and they jumped right in and said, "Oh, I know what you mean. That happened to me." And suddenly they've taken the floor, and you're listening to their experience. Your goal is to never do that to someone else, no matter if it's your employee, colleague, or even friend or family member. However, it's not that easy. In every conversation, you'll be doing what I refer to as the Brain On! internal dance. You'll be Brain On! for a few seconds, listening intently, focused on that person or email request, and then before you know it you find yourself thinking about something else or remembering a time when this happened to you. That is how our brains are built. But that is also why conversations can go astray or emotions get hijacked. By building your deep listening muscles in this station, you'll not only be able to be more present and attentive but also be more empathetic and compassionate in all your interactions.

How do you measure if you're building your listening muscle and becoming a strong listener? You can repeat what you've just heard or just read and are able to describe their underlying feelings associated with what is being asked or discussed. This is the only way to ensure you have it right. You might say, "Let me just make sure I'm understanding the issue. ..." Or, "What I heard you say is ... Is that accurate?" After the conversation, you can also do a quick self-assessment, rating how well you listened and how many times you were emotionally triggered or brain off and where you interrupted or pre-emptively jumped in with an answer or an opinion.

Check-in Station #4

Am I Brain On! during difficult conversations?

Jeremy Hunter, founding director of the Executive Mind Leadership Institute and professor of practice at the Peter F. Drucker Graduate School of Management, says that difficult conversations aren't what is difficult. It's the stories, thoughts, and beliefs we have about those conversations that make them so scary, dreadful, difficult, and frustrating. The first exercise in this station, even before you are about to have that difficult conversation, is to picture the outcome and envision how you want that meeting to go. You never know and can't control how the other person is going to respond, and that uncertainty alone can be a trigger for leaders. Preparing ahead of time and holding on to that vision of how you want to show up and what outcomes you want will have you stay on course and mentally strong during the meeting.

Checking in with yourself throughout the conversation is

critical—notice if you are getting tense or showing frustration or hesitation. That is your cue you've been triggered. The second most critical exercise during a difficult conversation is to pause before saying anything. And then third, don't try to anticipate or assume what the other person is thinking—instead, listen. This station is really a culmination of the previous check-ins and puts them together as a three-step routine to strengthen your resilience and your navigation of this very difficult, challenging situation.

There's no avoiding difficult conversations, but as a leader, remember that these dialogues can be essential for that individual's growth as well as the success of the organization. Your goal is to become highly skilled and emotionally strong at navigating difficult conversations.

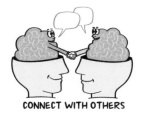

CONNECT WITH OTHERS

Check-in Station #5

Am I showing vulnerability and compassion as a leader?

In the new human-centric world of business, vulnerability and compassion are the best skills a leader can acquire. Compassion is something we must practice and cultivate; it is not something we are born with. That's why it's a mental fitness exercise, and it starts with the inner game. Before you can show compassion for others, you need to have self-compassion first. Many leaders tend to be self-critical on the way up the ladder, and self-compassion is one of the hardest things to learn.

Showing compassion for others as a leader is the willingness to empathize with an individual on your team and to recognize their inner challenges. The second part of showing compassion as a leader is to take some type of action to support that person. It's coming up with a couple of ways to help on an external level. It's asking, "Is there anything I can do to help support you?" It might mean bringing in benefits and resources that the organization offers or suggesting a specific training class.

Vulnerability is part of showing your team that you are human. It can be as simple as saying to your team, "I don't know" or "I was wrong on this one." It can even be a personal experience. That makes you a more "human" leader. I make it a point to share when I know I'm brain off and dealing with a personal problem, such as when someone in my family is sick or I'm dealing with a health crisis. Over time, they feel comfortable sharing, and, in the end, we learn from each other, which builds stronger relationships on and off the "playing field."

Check-in Station #6

Do I have a growth mindset for myself and my team?

Having autonomy, mastery, and purpose are the keys to having a high level of career well-being. A Brain On! leader knows that both themselves and their team need to grow, or risk stagnation or even deterioration of performance. If there are too many days where you and your team are just focused on tasks, this will result in a low-energy environment. Growing can take many shapes and forms—it can be growing knowledge and skills but also experiences and relationships.

Daniel Pink in his book *Drive* explains that "human beings have an innate inner drive to be autonomous, self-determined, and connected to one another. And when that drive is liberated, people achieve more and live richer lives."

To stay energized at work, find ways to grow your passions, your purpose, and your strengths—individually as a leader and collectively as a team. Bring in outside speakers or read a book together and discuss. If you've learned something new that's changed your life, bring that forward to your team.

When people feel like you are invested in their growth and see you work on and overcome your struggles, they stay Brain On! and are more energized. That strengthens your relationship with them, which strengthens the organization and its success.

Measuring Your Progress

Practicing the Brain On! Leadership Training Circuit daily by incorporating these check-ins into your workday can serve as a type of measurement of your leadership mental fitness score. Did you model Brain On! behavior before that meeting? How would you rate your listening skills today? Did you help anyone stay Brain On! based on how you handle a difficult conversation or challenging situation? Did you learn something new today? How did that affect your team's energy level?

Being a leader who people respect and want to work with starts by being a leader who has a good relationship with their own brain. A wise leader understands how to emotionally regulate themselves to keep their thinking Brain On! to avoid triggering others. All the leadership and management training in the world can't overcome a brain that is offline most of the time and not upgraded. Manage your own inner game first and see how far you and your team go.

LEADER HIGHLIGHT REEL

- Set the right tone as a leader. How you show up emotionally as a leader can be more impactful to employees than pay, promotions, or perks.

- Your emotions are contagious. The actions you take and words you choose are never neutral. You can either help remove barriers and obstacles in people's workdays or create more of them. You are responsible for keeping your team Brain On! by eliminating any work triggers and helping to avoid hijacking their emotions. This will ultimately determine if they have an energizing day instead of feeling burned out, disengaged.

- Check in with yourself throughout the day. A leader's main task throughout the day is to consciously and consistently check in to see if they are Brain On! in every interaction with another person. Do you feel distracted, tired, frustrated, or even angry? If so, take a break and get your brain back online. Any negative or fear-based emotion can trigger employees into a brain-off mode at any time.

BE A TEAM CAPTAIN BY INCORPORATING YOUR LEADERSHIP TRAINING CIRCUIT INTO EACH WORKDAY:

C – Check-in

A – Align with your Strengths

P – Pause

T – Talk Less; Listen More

A – Acknowledge and Recognize

I – Initiate Growth

N – Navigate the Difficult Conversations

Remember the Brain On! motto for leaders:

Learn it. Live it. Lead it.

CHAPTER 10
HR AS THE BRAIN ON! OWNER

"How do I energize our organization's collective brain?"

For the HR professionals whose role it is to focus on the people experience in an organization, I give a deep bow of appreciation and gratitude for all you do. Not many people realize how emotionally challenging your role is each day. Your responsibility is to ensure each person within your workplace family has everything they need to stay Brain On!, energized, and engaged. That is no easy feat. In fact, in this knowledge worker and transformative era, Human Resources, at its core, is about "Brain" Resource Management to best support the whole human. HR must ensure obstacles are removed and people have what they need to think, act, and be at their best every day at work. After working with hundreds of HR thought leaders over the years, I know that you are among the unsung heroes in the world. You are really the community builders, teachers, and caregivers of your organization, on the frontline supporting the health and welfare of your employees and setting the foundation for whether individuals survive or thrive in your organization.

Like the leaders of teams, your HR department has a designated role to play on the field each day—you are the creators, owners, and implementors of the mental fitness training playbook for an organization. It starts with you! Every brain in your organization is impacted by the programs, policies, benefits, training, and resources that HR develops and manages. In this chapter, I want to help ensure that anyone involved in HR knows the principles and actions needed to keep their workforce Brain On! and in an Energizer state to combat the rampant burnout, stress, and the effects of a potentially negative or toxic culture or team environment.

Quick disclaimer: I'm choosing to use HR as the common terminology because from my perspective, it doesn't matter as much what your department is called, but rather how your department operates. I'm using HR to refer to putting people first, being human-centric, deploying human design thinking, whole person systems, and life-work integration—the recognition that work is a critical component of a fulfilling life. Whether you have a title of People Operations, Chief People Officer, Total Reward, Human Resources, or Whole-Human Resources, it is fine if the underlying mission, purpose, and supportive actions are there. Similarly, whether you refer to your workforce as employees, team members, associates, or work family members is also irrelevant when you capture the essence of what an individual means to your organization and bring that forward in everything you do. What is important is that your philosophy and people approach is abundantly clear to each individual and always sincerely felt. These titles and "words" alone can help ensure your people feel cared for and Brain On!

As a unit, HR is responsible for developing and cultivating a positive employee experience each day. For years, the framework for doing so has been recognized and highlighted through organizational awards, based on engagement criteria such as:

- "My company values and recognizes my contribution."
- "I understand the vision and mission of the organization."
- "I have confidence in the leaders at my company."
- "My organization puts my well-being first."

But for organizations to receive high marks and see these critical criteria come to life, employees must first understand how they are wired as humans to improve their performance, how they can better emotionally regulate themselves, and what makes them feel compassionately connected and supported to their team. These are the Brain On! skills that HR must help employees and leaders build as a foundation for developing the energizing, high-functioning daily habits necessary to transform people's workday. *Without teaching these Brain On! skills, an organization is really leaving their employee engagement, leadership excellence, and its health and success to chance.*

How do you as an HR professional create a Brain On! employee experience? Overall, there are four key steps that will help you transform the way people work and create more energizing days:

Step 1: Initiate Brain On! for the organization

The HR department needs to first buy into its role as the "coach" or owner of the Brain On! approach on behalf of and in service to every single person in the organization and get leadership buy-in. The entire department needs to agree that this is its mode of operation, and the foundational framework for everything they create and support. Otherwise, the game is over before your players i.e., workforce, have assembled on the field, or in this case started their workday. Burnout, stress, low engagement, and turnover will continue to plague performance and organizational results.

Too often, each HR department or initiative has its own tasks, goals, and objectives, and may only come together in an all-team meeting once a month to discuss high-level projects and share what each group is working on. What I'm suggesting here is a more robust and integrated HR strategy where everyone is marching to the same drum, using the same approach, and operating from the same tenets with the same goals. Companies that have adopted the Brain On! approach often move to a master project plan and communications calendar centered on the employee experience. Projects are defined and scoped out by the employee action, behavior, or journey and not by the specific department or deliverable. The team calendar is built to aggregate and reflect every single communication, task, or opportunity that touches any employee during the month versus listing the items out by each department.

By having this clear picture of the employee experience that month, the HR team can then tailor its deadlines and communications to be more integrated and more rewards-centric instead of siloed, transactional, and triggering. Even if it is a difficult or complex message (like launching a new learning management or payroll system or conducting an active annual enrollment), providing a holistic, integrated view of what that employee needs to do and what that experience will look like that day, week, or month provides the certainty and clarity that employees need to feel cared for in a Brain On! way.

Step 2: Infuse Brain On! throughout HR decisions

In the beginning of this part of the book, I outlined some of the obstacles that get thrown in front of employees by HR—unintentionally, of course! Your goal is to ensure none of these obstacles as well as other potential ones get in the way of people having a Brain On! and energized day. To do so, HR must be aware of embedding the Brain On! approach in strategic decisions such as:

- How you attract, retain, and care for employees.
- The products and services that HR offers.
- The required leadership skills and people responsibilities.
- The organizational brand and reputation across all stakeholders and customers.
- Company innovations, products, and results.
- Contributions to the community and to the world.

How do you know if you've successfully delivered on these using a Brain On! approach? Before you hit send on a companywide communication or officially launch a new initiative, activate the purposeful pause as a team exercise, and ask questions such as, "Is the message clear or will it trigger uncertainty?" "Will this strengthen the organization's relationship with the employee?" "Will it be received as a reward or will it be perceived as a threat, unfair or unequal to certain groups, and elicit a brain-off, fear-based response and reaction?" This strategy, the purposeful pause, is a critical one that will help ensure HR is known for providing valuable resources and rewards, not threats or triggers.

You can also assess how Brain On! your actions are by using deep listening skills and paying attention to the subtle shifts in the attitudes or responses of people. Do employees or leaders email HR to complain or voice their concern about an announcement or communication you've recently sent? That means you've triggered their brains to go offline. You've unintentionally emotionally hijacked the people in your organization with your message, direction, or initiative, and they aren't thinking or operating as their best selves during that time. You can also monitor how serious an obstacle is by the number of people who didn't act or missed a critical deadline on something like annual enrollment or compliance training. It's often not that the initiative or change shouldn't be introduced, but how it is communicated and perceived, either as a reward or threat. You'll notice that threats as a collective will create anger, frustration, inaction, immobility, or rigidity. Rewards will create the movement forward or the action or behavior you want to see.

Step 3: Provide brain training for all employees

As the owner, implementor, and coach of Brain On!, the HR team's role is to build up people's mental strength and well-being. This requires supporting each employee with the appropriate education, tools, and resources to help them understand how their brain works and how to optimize and harness that power. Steps one and two build your operational foundation, but step three is where your approach really comes to life. Having Brain On! knowledge and skills will transform their employee experience and energize their days.

What does Brain On! training look like? The old approach is lunch-and-learns or one-time trainings on emotional intelligence for managers. Or perhaps you offer certain types of personality and behavioral assessments like Myers–Briggs, DiSC, or Gallup Strengths to high-potentials or leaders. These are all very useful and a great start, but I find these trainings and assessments are often one-and-done, very high-level, and never fully incorporated into people's performance goals and daily interactions and conversations. I also found they are typically only offered to a small set of employees. Expanding these types of assessments and training to all people will elevate and upgrade the entire organization to becoming Brain On! The new Brain On! approach to training has many levels to it and is continuously building skills that are embedded in daily operations, meetings, or job tasks. The goal is to train as much of your workforce as possible on how their brains are wired and how to build mental strength.

One of the questions I get asked is "how do I help reduce the stress of our employees?" Many organizations have offered one or two lunch-and-learns on stress management, but again, this does little to train and strengthen the collective brain and build good, lifelong habits. To create a Brain On! workplace that is high-functioning and resilient, the HR department should focus on expanding and incorporating ongoing training classes and tools that are geared toward and tied to reducing stress and making the workday more energizing for employees. Some examples of Brain On! training initiatives include growth mindset programs, unconscious bias skills, and mindfulness training. The key, whether building this in house or using a vendor partner, is to offer a wide range of brain optimization topics and trainings as multi-level courses (basic to advance) year-round that are inclusively designed for all learning styles (auditory, visual, and kinesthetic) and delivered through various mediums (print, video, web, app, live training, audio) in bite-sized, easy-to-digest formats.

For example, my employer, NFP, partners with a mental fitness vendor who offers a robust video training library, ready-to-send employee communications, and a mobile app for daily practice. Classes run in twelve-week blocks where we focus on one skill (i.e., conquering distraction and feelings of being overwhelmed at work) each quarter. They are offered to all global employees through a thirty-minute live, virtual training a couple times during the week. In addition, there is an app for employees that has the daily practices and meditations to go along with that topic. In the end, after twelve weeks we've learned how our brain operates in that work situation. We also know and can practice the skills to build that important mental muscle and good habits while also forming a stronger internal community by learning and exercising together.

To measure the impact and efficacy of your training efforts, it's important to remember that mental well-being is a subjective measurement, and only the employee themselves can determine if they feel Brain On! and are having an Energizer day. Their feedback is ultimately the best way to determine how successful your initiatives are in strengthening their brains and relationships at work. Quick informal pulse surveys before and after each class can help measure the effectiveness of each training session. Simply asking them to rate their stress level at the start of class (1-low to 5-high) and then doing so after the training most likely will demonstrate an immediate decrease in stress and anxiety. We found almost everyone reports those types of impactful results after each thirty minutes of practice. This leads to higher productivity and performance from that employee for the remainder of that workday. Win-win.

You can also survey class participants at four weeks and eight weeks after that segment ended to gauge if they are still practicing and applying their learnings and if they are still feeling less stressed. Make sure to include an open comment box in any survey and ask for any success stories and examples that you can use in your future communications to get more people interested and participating. Finally, vendor reports on utilization of the app or any technology used is also very helpful when determining the success of your program.

Step 4: Individualize Brain On! for each HR team

I'm encouraging HR teams to emotionally regulate themselves each day while they also emotionally regulate an entire organization.

A tall order, I understand. But the Brain On! quality of each department's decisions, communications, and conversations has the largest organizational impact on creating a culture of care and mental well-being. Below are some suggestions on how to individualize Brain On! for each HR team:

 ### LEARNING & DEVELOPMENT

This is listed first because L&D has the biggest role in transforming an organization to be Brain On! Personal development stops at about age eighteen in our society. We are never really taught how to be an adult and how to show up compassionately, maturely, and generously, especially at work. We aren't ever taught how our brains learn, work to perform our jobs, and interact with others on teams. We aren't given an instruction manual on how to regulate our emotions, or the business and personal impact of not being aware of our emotions and effectively processing them. Those "learning gaps" are the challenges that HR Learning & Development needs to own and take on for the mental well-being and future success of the organization.

The HR Learning & Development department is the executive champion for ensuring the entire workforce and organization works in a more productive, sustainable, and regenerative way. Understanding how our brains work, how collective brains work together, and how to train brains for better focus, productivity, time management, conversation, and communications are all adult development trainings and skills. I've found that thriving organizations who put people in the center of their culture have well-being initiatives primarily under and owned by HR Learning & Development. Your team should act as the curriculum designer for everything both employees and leaders need to know to be Brain On! and energized at work. Developing each person to be a mentally strong, high-performing, collaborative employee is a business imperative for your department.

Your Brain On! role is to design an overall curriculum and offering that ensures personal mastery, including emotional intelligence, unconscious bias, focus and attention training, self-awareness, having difficult conversations, and effective interpersonal skills. I've also found that to be successful in training the collective brains, HR Learning & Development teams still need to work closely with your Talent, Benefits, and Diversity, Equity, Inclusion, and Belonging colleagues. The goals and initiatives of these departments will overlap in terms of creating a psychologically safe and inclusive culture. Organizational success will be determined by the depth, breadth, and commitment level of the mental fitness training offering and participation at all levels. That is why an integrated HR approach, led by L&D, is needed to transform the workplace now and in the future.

 ## RECRUITMENT

Attracting key talent is just like scouting for the best players on a sports team. Or reviewing and interviewing applicants for a top school. You have the responsibility to bring forward and hire the best and brightest, which is no longer just about work skills and achievements. You want to look for people who display these Brain On! interpersonal skills we've been discussing and are open to the Brain On! approach to continue to transform and energize your entire workforce, especially at the manager and leader level.

As the "first face and brain" of the organization, the one-on-ones you have with potential hires can either create a reward or obstacle about joining the organization (first impressions matter). It's essential you practice your Brain On! skills, especially some of the more human or "soft skills" that are becoming more critical in the recruiting role, such as curiosity, deep listening, and empathy. And let me be clear—soft skills are a misnomer. These aren't easy skills to learn and develop, and they take as much time, effort, focus, and practice as running and managing your recruitment processes and systems and sourcing your candidate pool.

 ## TALENT

There are so many key initiatives that a Talent department manages where the Brain On! approach can make or break the success of the employee experience:

- **Onboarding.** This is when Talent serves as the Brain On! Ambassador of the organization to successfully set up new employees right from the start. There is nothing scarier for a new employee than the first few days at a new job. The brain's amygdala is on hyperalert, and new beliefs and stories will form quickly. Introducing new employees to the

Brain On! approach by teaching these skills and strategies during New Hire Orientation and their first few days on the job would be a great first assignment.

- **First Ninety Days skills training.** However long your onboarding period (thirty, sixty, preferably ninety days), strategically train new employees on Brain On! skills throughout this critical and "brain-sensitive" time frame. Teach them how their brain works in this new situation and what to look out for, how to build stronger connections with their new team members and colleagues, and ensure their strengths are communicated to their manager so they can be incorporated into the initial goal-setting and job-responsibility discussions.

- **Performance planning and reviews.** We've already discussed how setting goals can trigger people's brains off. Ensuring an employee's goals are tied to their strengths and well-being is critical when performance planning time comes. When reviewing and providing feedback on those goals, many companies are eliminating annual reviews because capturing an entire year's worth of work results and areas to improve is often overwhelming and counterproductive. It often turns off an employee's brain to go back through a year's worth of effort. Just like goal setting can turn a brain-off, annual performance reviews usually have this effect on individuals as well. Teach leaders how and why these performance discussions can be one of the biggest triggers for employees and how to ensure these conversations are structured to keep Brains On.

Encourage recognition and carefully crafted constructive feedback throughout the year to energize people and provide certainty regarding their job performance. This is what will keep an employee's brain from being hijacked with worry and enhances their feeling of being cared for and appreciated – Brain On!

- **Training on difficult conversations.** Partner with Learning & Development to provide all talent with the skill set to not only navigate ongoing performance discussions but also difficult conversations. Both the leaders and employees need to be armed with these skills to successfully navigate any internal or external challenging conversation. Developing a culture where constructive feedback can be given without emotional backlash provides the psychological safety and transparency that is the mark of a thriving and mentally strong organization.

 ## COMPENSATION

Compensation represents the biggest and most frequent "reward" an employee's brain receives from the organization. However, pay can also be the biggest obstacle or perceived threat as well, creating a lens of negativity from which their job and employer is viewed. When compensation triggers brains-off, HR and leaders will hear things like "I'm not paid fairly." "I can make more money doing the same job at ABC company." And internally, individuals are thinking even more damaging thoughts, when brain-off, such as, "I can't believe I'm paid so little for all the work I do." "I'm doing the work of two people."

"My company doesn't recognize my worth." Resentment from this brain-off thinking will accumulate. and it will be hard to overcome and get them to be Brain On! again.

In today's world, most people don't experience any visible reward associated with their hard work except maybe annually during the salary or performance review meeting. Their hard-earned money goes out as fast as it comes in due to automatic payroll deposit and online bill payments depleting the account faster than the time it takes to see their bank account increase with the paycheck in it. This process has left employees brains-off. Without this visible reward mechanism (payday acknowledgement and celebration), employees default to a threat state (out of sight, out of mind), questioning their pay, their value, and if it's worth all the stress and work they put forth. A Compensation team with a Brain On! approach recognizes each payday as an opportunity to communicate value, recognition, appreciation, and rewards to employees through creative communications, intranet postings, calendar reminders, reflection exercises, and financial well-being initiatives.

One company sends out an easy emoji pulse survey (happy, sad, angry) every payday, asking just one question "Do you feel you were paid fairly for your work and results these last two weeks?" Thumbs up or thumbs down is indicated along with an open comment box allowing them to elaborate on their answer. There are two wins here. First, by asking people to reflect on their work and pay every two weeks, it gives them clarity and perspective on their contribution and value. Secondly, it demonstrates to the employee that the employer cares about them. And, by the way, you'd be surprised, but there were mostly thumbs-up responses and great appreciation for this activity.

 BENEFITS

The Benefits department is the primary caregiver of your workforce by providing solutions to boost energy and motivation (that's why it's part of Total Rewards). My experience, however, is that many Benefits products and services are fear-based (you won't have enough money for retirement, miss an enrollment deadline and you won't receive health care, etc.) And to employees, the Benefits department is full of scary must-dos and potential downfalls that trigger employees' brains to go offline.

When marketing and communicating these benefits, 99 percent of the time you must assume brains will be turned off by whatever you are announcing, even if it's an important and helpful new benefit, such as long-term care, that is intended to better their life or financial position. Think about how annual enrollment goes for employees. Every year across the globe, employees wonder and ask only two things once annual enrollment starts. How much are you increasing my premiums? And what are you taking away this year? Just seeing the words "annual enrollment" signals alarm bells. People usually wait until the last day to make changes because they find the process confusing, scary, frustrating, and overwhelming. No one wants to think about how sick they will get during the upcoming year, how many prescriptions they will need, or how much money is needed to survive if they or their partner dies next year. Yikes! No wonder a person's brain is triggered off, and they can't make any decision or the right decision.

Even the new shiny pennies or "wins" you are introducing during annual enrollment can trigger people's brains off. You might say you are offering a $200 well-being credit for anyone that gets an annual physical or completes a quarterly health activity challenge, such as steps tracking or eating healthy. However, only the people doing that currently— the active and healthy brains— stay on. Most brains are triggered immediately off in fear, just thinking about having to give up their favorite sugary drink/snack, getting poked with a needle for biometrics reporting, or having to now find time to exercise or switch to the exercise being promoted. And these immediate brain-off reaction examples are just related to the benefits election process. During the year, any situation or event when the employee now uses your products (like group medical insurance) usually involves a scary, stressful, brain-off situation each time, other than maybe having a baby, and therefore continuously reinforces their fears associated with Benefits.

There are so many more examples, but the point here is that all your hard work in curating an amazing benefit offering for the good of your employees immediately and consistently triggers or keeps brains off. Which is why utilization may be low, consumerism isn't taking hold, emergency rooms continue to serve as primary care doctors, and why many people continue to only seek care when a medical crisis occurs.

Given annual enrollment is your time to really shine and interact with employees, here are some tips on how to make the experience more Brain On!

- Use human-centered design thinking and neuromarketing techniques to develop out-of-the-box communications, such as engaging benefits guides. Few organizations have updated their benefits guides in years, and most are not intuitive or user-friendly. Adding examples and stories of individuals representing your demographics helps people relate. Including icons like a money sign next to benefits that can save them money, such as their Health Savings Accounts or Dependent Day Care accounts, are very helpful in turning brains back on and hopefully taking advantage of these offerings. Even ensuring your entire total rewards offering is in one place on a mobile app, not just a partial listing on an intranet or benefits enrollment system, allows them to easily find everything they need 24/7 and elicit the support of their partner when making these important decisions.

- Offer an off-cycle annual enrollment for voluntary or lifestyle benefits outside of your core ERISA plans. Pick three or four of these and carve them out of the annual election process so employees can spend the additional time building more knowledge, confidence, and consumerism around these products as well as reducing their threat response associated with having too many costly choices during annual enrollment. I've seen much more uptake and enrollment success when employers dedicate a month to a certain benefit, such as critical illness, long-term care, or caregiving solutions, and start training them on one topic at a time. By doing so, you'll keep employees Brains On! and feel rewarded by giving employees the confidence to make rational, appropriate decisions one-by-one. Time Out! Let's check in. Did I trigger your brain off with this suggestion of adding more benefit enrollments to your year? If so, take three deep breaths. It may sound like a lot of work, but it isn't, especially if you enlist your broker and carrier to help develop the communications and training and use a benefits enrollment solution to ensure employees get answers to their questions and assistance to make their elections.

- Partner with Learning & Development to offer Benefits 101 trainings ahead of annual enrollment season (preferably year-round) that include decision support assessments, videos, tools, and benefits calculators. This teaches employees how to be a smart consumer and a champion of their physical, financial, and mental well-being. The goal here is to put the benefits back into Benefits. Building individual expertise and confidence through skills training will help move your fear-based (brain-off) offerings to truly the rewards-based (Brain On!) offerings they are intended to be.

 ## DIVERSITY, EQUITY, INCLUSION, AND BELONGING (DEIB)

Every single aspect of DEIB is a Brain On! mental fitness

exercise that requires training, practice, and skill building daily and throughout a person's career. We are wired to live in social groups, but we aren't wired to easily build relationships or make sure they are healthy ones defined by respect for individual differences and needs.

Anyone that is different from us can subconsciously trigger our brains off. Mitigating bias, suspending judgment, seeing the commonality versus the differences, being an ally of others, and showing up with compassion are all key aspects and focuses of a Brain On! approach. Training leaders and employees to be aware of and remove the daily obstacles that cause strife, tension, stress, and negativity is of the highest priority for an organization to protect its culture, brand, and reputation.

DEIB is about rewiring our old habits, patterns, behaviors, and thoughts. This takes significant time, dedication, and training of all individuals to really upgrade the collective brain to be open minded and inclusive. And why it's important for the DEIB team to coordinate and work with Learning & Development on these skills-building classes. Here are some DEIB training tips:

- **Help all employees understand how their brains are wired for bias and that it is completely normal.** There can be shame and self-loathing when people think they should know better or act better or didn't know a certain fact. There can also be a lot of fear holding people back from connecting with someone else, worried about doing or saying the wrong thing. Helping people understand how their brains are wired for bias and then the things they can do to upgrade their brains through training and practice should be reinforced many times throughout as many opportunities as possible.

- **Unconscious bias training needs to be more than one or two sessions.** That will never be enough to rewire people's brains and ingrain these important habits. Incorporating bias mitigation into all Learning & Development trainings to develop communication, conversations, and decision-making skills is key. Start with a Brain ON audit, by reviewing all employee trainings offered that are outside of an individual job performance skill set and imbed a part about what bias might show up in this topic, how to become Brain On! and mitigate that bias using mental fitness exercises (found in chapter 7), examples, and group discussions.

- **Incorporating and ensuring your DEIB initiatives are a core pillar of your well-being program is critical.** If someone doesn't feel seen, heard, or included, that means their brains are off and they are operating from a threatened or fear state and experiencing the physiological impact of that stress response in their bodies and mind. They will be less likely to participate in meetings or be fully engaged in their work. Feeling a strong sense of belonging within an organization is the foundation of a person's well-being at work. Incorporate community building, empathy, allyship, and diversity of thought into your well-being programs and incentive design. The easiest place to start is establishing internal online forums or communities. These are sometimes referred to as Employee Resource Groups, Infinity Groups, etc. Sharing experiences, holding education sessions, or recognizing holidays for that specific resource group can help build compassion and community. Incorporating attendance of these events into your well-being points program is an easy way to include DEIB mental fitness training into your overall well-being initiatives.

HR BRAIN ON! FRAMEWORK

HR benefits and programs typically represent one of the largest, if not the largest, expense for any organization. HR is often considered one big cost center, unintentionally triggering a brain-off attitude among the C-Suite and board of directors. A Brain On! approach to HR can turn this perception around, by focusing on the positive impact its teams play in creating a more productive workforce and a culture that attracts the best talent. Keep this HR Brain On! Framework close at hand for discussions with upper management about the role of HR in employee engagement, productivity, and performance results. Let this serve as a highlight reel in chart format as you prioritize the well-being of your organization and its people.

HR's Department	Brain-off HR	Brain On! HR
HR's financial role	Cost center	Investment center
HR's delivery model	Siloed	Integrated
HR's function	Business support	Business value
HR's purpose	Attract and retain	Attract, retain, and care for
HR's expertise	Total rewards, professional development, diversity and equity	Human performance, energy management, the employee experience
HR's business contribution	Creating a high-performing organization	Create a high-performing organization that is mentally strong and healthy
Employee experience model	Centered around the job role and tasks	Centered around meaning, contribution, belonging, and well-being
Career well-being model	Based on job skill acquisition, pay, and promotions	Based on autonomy, mastery, purpose, recognition, and relatedness
Culture model	Business solutions, services, and results is the glue that connects and unites teams	Human connection, relatedness, collaboration, compassion, and belonging is the glue that connects people, and emotional intelligence is the language that unites the workforce

Employee's Perspective	Brain-off HR	Brain On! HR
Learning and development	Job skills training	Life skills, job skills, brain optimization skills; holistic adult development
Talent	Performance monitored and measured through SMART goals. Annual feedback and recognition based on output and results	Performance monitored and measured through alignment to strengths-based, SMART-ER goals. Ongoing 360-degree feedback and recognition based on output and results
Compensation	Scarcity-mentality, controlling costs	Prosperity-mentality, creating financial freedom
Benefits	Fear-based, risk-mitigation products and policies	Rewards-based; life-enhancing products and policies
Diversity, Equity, Inclusion and Belonging	Standard metrics and targets (diversity of workforce; pay equity)	Broader people-focused metrics (connectedness, inclusion, and equitable pay, benefits, promotions, and rewards)

By integrating all HR functions and deliverables around keeping brains on and energized, you transform the employee experience from burnout and stress to resilience and growth, from surviving to thriving, and from meaningless to meaningful. A Brain On! organization can put the human back into all aspects of Human Resources by upgrading the collective brain.

CHAPTER 11

BECOMING A BRAIN ON! REGENERATIVE CULTURE

"How can my organization really come alive?"

There's nothing more thrilling for me than to see people in an organization really working together to dream bigger and go further than they ever imagined. You can feel the electricity flowing through every project and department. Everyone is filled with a positive energy that is contagious. Everyone feels so alive!

A Brain On! Regenerative organization is the culmination and visible results of your entire workforce operating as their best selves through continually upgrading the greatest "technology" an organization has—its collective brain. In regenerative agriculture, the farmers help the land become more biodiverse and productive every year. The same concept applies to your work environment and culture—an organization consciously and intentionally helps people improve their skills, productivity, and overall lives. I've been greatly influenced in my Brain On! regenerative approach by David Rock, co-founder and CEO of the NeuroLeadership Institute, who has been a pioneer in the notion that an organization should leave people better off day after day, year after year. His path to a Regenerative organization focuses on having a growth mindset, among other components.

The Brain On! approach takes Dr. Rock's thinking one step further—its core principle is that mental well-being is the foundation upon which the other elements of a regenerative culture must be built. Every employee must understand their emotional triggers and monitor for daily obstacles, while leaders and HR teams carefully assess their own interactions and communications to not add to these triggers and obstacles, but consciously model and contribute to making it a healthier and happier work environment and workday. Employees, Leaders, and HR teams should all be an additive positive force to the "soil" or work environment and workday (#BetterTogether!).

Why set the goal to become a Brain On! Regenerative organization? It's because every decision, communication, and action in your organization originates from the brains behind your operations— your people. If their brains are off, your business is off. And because of that, a Brain On! Regenerative workplace is the only kind of organization that will successfully handle the uncertainty, complexity, and change that is inevitable in the future. I've consistently observed that the root cause of an organization's issues with low engagement, burnout, high turnover, pay disparity, and many other challenges is that people are brain off most of the time—or "below the line" as we learned. That's why my manifesto at this stage of my executive career is this: *I believe that the quality and success of an organization is primarily dependent on having a Brain On! workforce.*

Let's look at what a Brain On! Regenerative organization is compared to other types of organizations by adapting our individual Energizer model from Chapter 4:

THE BRAIN ON! ORGANIZATIONAL MATRIX

ORGANIZATION
BRAIN ON!

Sustainable   Regenerative

DISENGAGED   HIGHLY ENGAGED
WORKFORCE   WORKFORCE

Transactional   Depletive

ORGANIZATION
BRAIN OFF

TRANSACTIONAL

This is an organization that has no heartbeat. It doesn't provide more meaning beyond the daily tasks. It may run smoothly but has this emptiness feeling or shell, just doesn't feel alive. It's the exact opposite of "coming alive" and regenerative. What I see with this type of organization is the employer-employee relationship is very black and white—"you do this, you get paid that." Some refer to this as a command-and-control organization. There is little meaningful exchange between management and employees. Benefits and pay are not tied to an organizational mission and are stripped down to the basics. The culture carries strong overtones of being risk averse, often grounded in old patterns and ways of thinking (fixed mindset, brain off), and not progressive. The same procedures and operations have been in place for years. Employees are not engaged because they don't feel recognized or cared for as a human being. Leaders in these transactional organizations or even operating in a transactional mode display a lack of emotional intelligence and commitment to "people-first" and their mental well-being.

DEPLETIVE

This is when the brains in the organization are operating offline, but productivity is high. This happens when the organization takes, takes, takes, and continues to ask of people well beyond their capacity, and offers only their total rewards package in return. A depletive organization also tends to do more with less, pay isn't equitable, and recognition isn't consistent or meaningful. This leads to a toxic culture where employees feel burned out, overwhelmed, and run ragged. Organizations in fast-moving industries such as retail, financial services, technology, healthcare, and the military, as well as newer businesses, such as start-ups, can often operate in a depletive mode. Also, organizations that have extended busy seasons lasting a good part of the year, with no built-in recovery time or restorative practices, fall into this quadrant as well. In a depletive mode, the work may be aligned with an individual's passion (which is why it's listed toward high engagement potential), but the work structure and work environment are taxing on their health and well-being. Causing them to work in survival, brain-off mode just to make it through the day (just like in the Chapter 4 quadrant for the individual). In the long run, an organization pays for it with an unhealthier workforce, lower engagement, higher attrition, more costly errors and issues, less collaboration, and a lack of innovation.

SUSTAINABLE

This is what most organizations today have been led to believe is the "gold standard." They don't know that there is something more powerful and inspiring. That there is a better way to design the workday. That there is a new Brain On! approach that takes employees to a better place than just sustainable with good results, good relationships with employees. A sustainable organization is an "okay" place to be because it has a neutral or "net zero" impact on an employee. It has adopted the "right" people mindset and measurements such as engagement and retention. But much of their employee communications and actions are hit-and-miss when it comes to truly engaging and energizing their workforce over the long run.

For example, the organization does not heavily invest in nor is it firmly grounded in innovation, total rewards, or having a broader impact in society. The decision framework is still heavily slanted toward business outcomes over people outcomes, and the financial strategy defaults to applying any discretionary dollar to business needs instead of also considering investing in their people as the key to improving business results. These are the critical initiatives that get put on hold until next year or get bumped to the bottom of the priority list in favor of spending the money on a business need instead. I understand and am sympathetic to the pressure of the bottom line. My degree is in accounting, and I have worked at a large private firm managing million-dollar budgets and P&Ls. When I talk to CFOs and executives, they are appreciative of my ability to translate the business case of building a mentally strong organization and the return on value of implementing this approach. This initiative does not take money to implement. It simply takes an open mind and firm commitment from leadership to focus on upgrading the best "technology" and assets you'll ever have access to at your organization—the collective brain.

Sustainable organizations are missing the huge opportunity to fully engage and empower employees by not investing in people-first over business-first and aligning the organizational strengths and mission to the individual strengths.

REGENERATIVE

Becoming Regenerative is the highest standard that an organization can hold itself to. It's one that is committed to creating, maintaining, and upgrading the playing field and the work experience for employees so they are Brain On!, energized, and mentally strong to perform every day.

A Regenerative Brain On! organization is an inspiring place to be, where collaboration is natural, and performance is always improving for the teams and individuals. The organization helps employees see a clear path to the end zone or the finish line of that day, that quarter, and that year and helps them get there in a healthy, energized way. People understand the mission of the business, feel aligned, inspired, and included, and know how to move towards the goals in a more collaborative and restorative way. There's a positive and supportive Brain On! energy that empowers everyone, from the top leaders to the newest employee. There's a sense of pride in what the organization stands for both in business and in society. Every person understands the supportive rules for every interaction or meeting:

- It's okay to take a pause before speaking or answering an email to check in with one's emotional state to avoid triggering others.

- When someone on your team is acting brain-off, approach them with curiosity and compassionate inquiry to check in with their mental well-being.

- Acting as protectors and guardians of the Brain On! approach. This means helping each other get back up and online when things aren't going well. Managers promote and support time off from work or timeouts during the day for employees when necessary so they can rest and re-energize their brains.

I'm suggesting four principles that a Brain On! Regenerative organization should live by to enrich the working environment, strengthen its relationship with each employee, and create that ecosystem that empowers people to flourish.

PRINCIPLE #1: ADOPT A CARE CONTRACT

The old relationship between workers and the organization was very transactional. The employee was paid wages in return for a job completed. Then it evolved to attracting and retaining employees through rewards, primarily pay and a mix of benefits. However, this still didn't include an employee's well-being or their personal life at the forefront and as the foundation of the employment contract. It didn't go the extra mile in taking responsibility and care of the employee while working at the organization. The Regenerative Brain On! approach expands HR's typical philosophy to attract, retain, and care for talent, therefore transforming the benefits of working there into a "caring contract" that gives employees the emotional and psychological support they need. Some of this is accomplished operationally by doubling down on DEIB and removing biases and inequities and creating an integrative HR approach that makes the employee feel cared for with every interaction and experience with your offerings and resources. Some of this is found in the individual Brain Boosters we discussed in Chapter 8—programs that help an employee with self-care initiatives. And most importantly, by developing Brain On! leaders who are responsible for implementing this contract every day with those they manage. This care contract is the new manifestation of the employee experience.

PRINCIPLE #2: CENTER ON EMOTIONAL INTELLIGENCE

For employees to feel psychologically supported, connected, and valued, everyone needs to understand and be taught emotional self-mastery and regulation. These are the two core skills that need to be embedded in all learning and training modules. These are human skills that are on par with job skills as far as determining the success of an organization. At the organizational level, emotional intelligence also plays an important role. During your organization's crunch season or budget season, your workforce will feel more stress and burnout and can easily slip into brain-off mode. This is when more triggering events will happen with employees, resulting in more errors, issues, tension, and conflicts. This is the time to ensure your teams are constantly referring to this Organization Playbook and consistently practicing the mental fitness exercises we covered. The overarching measurement of a mentally strong and emotionally intelligent organization is that with each decision or communication it intentionally strengthens—not degrades—your connection to your employees.

PRINCIPLE #3: ENSURE TRIGGER-FREE COMMUNICATIONS

As you've learned by now, the wrong choice of words can trigger employees and shut down their brains in a nanosecond. The right words, on the other hand, spark the positive energy that can fuel an employee's day, quarter, and year. Whether your organization has an internal communications department, or the department or business leader is writing employee communications, their single focus must be on moving people toward the future in a positive and transparent way. Don't let employees hang in suspense, wondering what is going to happen. That triggers uncertainty, which is the last thing employees want to feel at work. Being specific and clear in your communication helps people process on a thinking level instead of emotional level. In addition, requesting continual employee feedback is a way of rewarding brains and keeping them energized and engaged in the company's mission and future direction.

PRINCIPLE #4: REWARD A GROWTH MINDSET

I spent a good chunk of time in Chapter 5 talking about the new strengths-based approach to goal setting for individuals. This type of goal setting succeeds within organizations because people have been encouraged—and expected—to have a growth mindset. To have thriving people, teams, and a successful business, an organization must reward having a growth mindset. As an organization, this reinforces the concept that is okay to fail if you look at it as a learning opportunity. Some companies even reward employees for failing "smart" and identifying their learnings to implement better processes based on this. Rewards are all used to keep employees Brain On! and excited about innovating and improving the company instead of being fearful or risk averse.

Brain On! Organizational Audit

The following Brain On! audit can help you assess how your organization and culture is activating these principles:

CARE ASSESSMENT

- Do leaders truly value employees, and do employees feel valued?
- Do people within the organization respect, support, and care about one another as people, not just as employees there to complete certain job tasks?
- Do the resources, programs, policies, and the environment support an employee's ability to thrive in all areas of well-being?
- Are employees provided the tools and resources they need to work safely and productively?
- Are employees encouraged and supported to be authentic and be themselves?
- Is recovery part of the workday?
- Are employees happy and proud to work here?

EMOTIONAL INTELLIGENCE ASSESSMENT

- Do people master their inner game before outer game?
- Do leaders and the work environment provide employees with autonomous support versus using incentives to drive behaviors?
- Are individuals encouraged to continuously upgrade their brain and work to become their best selves?

- Are interactions, decisions, and communications developed using the Brain On! approach?
- Is there purposeful pause or strategic silence built into the start of meetings, daily operations, high-stress days, or busy season?
- Is curiosity, compassion, and appreciative inquiry the foundation for discovery and understanding?

COMMUNICATIONS ASSESSMENT

- Are the mission, vision, and values clearly articulated? Does every employee know how they fit within them?
- Is there clear, timely, and meaningful communication for employees? Are employees encouraged to share ideas and feedback?
- Is accountability embraced? Are the rules clear and do they apply to everyone?
- Does the organizational language and words used strengthen the employee-employer relationship and the relationship between colleagues?

GROWTH ASSESSMENT

- Are employees empowered and enabled to leverage their strengths?
- Is ongoing feedback provided for employees in the spirit of ongoing growth and development versus simply measuring performance?
- Does the environment foster innovation, creativity, and meaningful work?
- Are people accomplishing what they desire with mastery and purpose?

- Is the growth mindset a foundation for learning?

The Regenerative Spirit Is Energizing

To borrow from Hollywood, a Regenerative Brain On! organization is one with the "it" factor. There's a somewhat elusive, but highly attractive, essence about the organization that you can get a hint of in your first interaction with the company but can only truly experience once you've worked within the culture for a time. It's how the people feel working with each other day in and day out. It's how they treat each other with care, compassion, collaboration, and connection. There's an immediate energy in the room when the meeting starts. Everyone feels like they belong; there's no subterfuge or hidden agendas. People finish their day more alive and filled up than when the day began.

In my years of working with hundreds of companies as an expert in well-being, what I have learned and seen time and time again is the root cause of people and performance issues is a brain-off way of working. Creating an organization that feels alive starts by committing to a Brain On! approach where we teach people how their brains work, how to build a better relationship with their brains, how to be self-aware to notice when they are brain off, and how to build the habits and skills to stay energized throughout the day.

This is fundamentally a new operating system for individuals and organizations that's human centered and human designed to rewire the way we think, the way we feel, and the way we work. Our future happiness and success as individuals, organizations, and society depends on capturing this regenerative energy and spirit. Brain On!

EPILOGUE
IT'S GO TIME! START WINNING THE WORKDAY

On your mark, get set . . . Brain On!

Congratulations. You made it to the end of the book with your trainer, and now possess a clear understanding of the importance of prioritizing mental well-being at work above everything else.

This foundational understanding of mental well-being and mental fitness exercises is just the beginning. The next challenge in front of you, whether you're an executive, an HR professional, or a trusted employee, is taking the knowledge you have gained and incorporating these strategies and practices into your workday and sharing these strategies and experiences with your colleagues and friends.

The opportunity I pose to you today–yes right now–is to flip the script and start winning your workday. The first step is ensuring you don't succumb to ineffective work habits you have grown accustomed to (i.e., operating brain off and on autopilot), by using the playbooks and mental fitness exercises we shared in the previous chapters.

When it comes to winning the workday, consistency and daily practice are everything. Every day, on the job, you will be faced with navigating the ever changing and challenging workday obstacle course, so the sooner you get started the better. The good news is you already know 90 percent of the grueling course you're facing—it's documented in your calendar and on your to-do list. The best news is that in order to strengthen your brain, you don't need specialized equipment, the latest workout gear, or anything other than a firm intention, positive attitude, and patience toward yourself to excel.

You can start right away.

Always keep in mind that our brains have never been upgraded since the beginning of time. Your habits are not going to change overnight and it's going to take a level of dedication on your part to upgrade your brain. The workplace provides countless opportunities to practice the skills you have learned and build mental strength.

Simply being aware if you are Brain On! or brain off throughout the day will go a long way toward achieving the results you seek. Show up with compassion, curiosity, and gratitude while remaining on task without being distracted. These are all traits that will strengthen your mental acuity and create immediate results and important wins when you do your daily exercises.

Also, remember: out of sight, out of mind. Meaning, *Brain On!* is a resource you should keep handy so you can access the information whenever it's needed. Anytime you are feeling angry, frustrated, or overwhelmed, and recognize the signals your brain may be offline and you need to recalibrate, *Brain On!* should be easily accessible and top of mind. It's your number one, on-the-job training resource moving forward.

This book will serve as your indispensable reminder and allow you to continuously check in with yourself and understand what's going on. Then you can reset, recharge, and get your Brain On!

As an organization, implementing an integrated HR approach and the Brain On! framework will give you a jump start in creating, enhancing, and supporting a brain-friendly environment. You're ready to cultivate a regenerative obstacle course filled with growth opportunities, connections, and high-functioning and rewarding experiences.

You are positioned for success. You now have all the tools and knowledge necessary to prioritize mental well-being and the strategies and skills necessary for winning the workday—today and tomorrow.

Brain On! Game On!
You've. Got. This.
Go out there and win that workday!

REFERENCES

These references helped shape my thinking of many of the concepts and insights about the brain I learned over the years. A big thank you to some of the psychologists, neuroscientists, physicians, researchers, and authors in my personal "brain trust" who guided me on my path to becoming your Brain Trainer:

1   Dr Evian Gordon, Founder and Chief Medical Officer at Total Brain, www.totalbrain.com/about-us.

2   Daniel Levitin, *The Organized Mind* (Penguin Press, 2015).

3   Dr. Nathaniel Kleitman, Professor Emeritus in the Department of Physiology at the University of Chicago, www.uchicagomedicine.org/forefront/news/nathaniel-kleitman-phd-1895-1999.

4   Dr. Jeffrey Schwartz, *Brain Lock* (HarperCollins, 1996).

5   Dr. Daniel Amen, *Change Your Brain, Change Your Life* (Crown, 1998).

6   Rick Hanson, *Hardwiring Happiness* (Harmony, 2013).

7   Dr. Dan Siegel, Clinical Professor of Psychiatry at the UCLA School of Medicine and founding Co-Director of the Mindful Awareness Research Center, drdansiegel.com/hand-model-of-the-brain.

8   Dr. David Rock, *Brain at Work* (Harper Business, 2009).

9   Greater Good Science Center, University of California-Berkeley, Faculty Director Dacher Keltner, greatergood.berkeley.edu/article/item/how_many_different_human_emotions_are_there.

10 Brené Brown, *Atlas of the Heart* (Random House, 2021).

11 Sharon Salzberg, Real Happiness at Work (Workman Publishing, 2013).

12 Dr. Amishi Jha, *Peak Mind* (HarperOne, 2021).

13 Carol Dweck, *Mindset* (Random House, 2006).

14 Gallup, "What Is Employee Engagement and How Do You Improve It?", www.gallup.com/workplace/285674/improve-employee-engagement-workplace.aspx.

15 Tom Rath, *Life's Greatest Question: Discover How You Contribute to the World* (Silicon Guild, 2020).

16 Marcia Wieder, *Dream, Clarify, and Create* (Next Century, 2016).

17 Gallup, "How to Set Goals (Then Achieve Them) Using CliftonStrengths," https://www.gallup.com/cliftonstrengths/en/358019/set-goals-using-your-strengths.aspx.

18 Shawn Achor and Michelle Gielan, "Consuming Negative News Can Make You Less Effective at Work," *Harvard Business Review*, September 14, 2015, https://hbr.org/2015/09/consuming-negative-news-can-make-you-less-effective-at-work.

19 Tony Schwartz, *The Way We're Working Isn't Working: The Four Forgotten Needs That Energize Great Performance* (Free Press, 2010).

20 Ellen Langer, *The Power of Mindful Learning,* (Da Capo, 1997).

21 Jim Dethmer, *The 15 Commitments of Conscious Leadership: A New Paradigm for Sustainable Success* (Conscious Leadership Group, 2015).

22 Dr. Darren Weissman, *Awakening to the Secret Code of Your Mind* (Hay House, 2010).

23 Janice Marturano, *Finding the Space to Lead: A Practical Guide to Mindful Leadership* (Bloomsbury Press, 2014).

24 Tara Brach, *Radical Compassion: Learning to Love Yourself and Your World with the Practice of RAIN* (Penguin Life, 2019).

25 Dr. Martin Seligman, Director of the Penn Positive Psychology Center, https://ppc.sas.upenn.edu/people/martin-ep-seligman.

26 Scott Shute, *The Full Body YES! Change Your Work and Your World from the Inside* Out (Page Two, 2021).

27 Dr. Dan Siegel, drdansiegel.com/healthy-mind-platter.

28 Daniel Pink, *A Whole New Mind* (Riverhead Books, 2005).

WITH GRATITUDE

I'm extremely grateful to so many people who have helped me over the years train my brain, build my mental strength expertise, and ultimately helped me realize my dream of authoring this book and sharing my insights and work with the world. This list of wonderful people and organizations is surely incomplete. I hope that others who have influenced my work and life that I have neglected to mention will forgive me in advance. Everyone should be so lucky as me to have such support from so many directions.

MY BOOK TEAM: First, this book wouldn't be possible without KN Literary Arts and my amazing and extremely talented collaborative writer, Melinda Cross, who magically brought my vision and decades of experience to life by remarkably translating my pages and pages of research, ideas, and thoughts into a meaningful treasure. In addition, I want to thank Tanmay Voya for his brilliant illustrations and visuals, which added such richness to the words. And a huge thank you to my extraordinary team at Amplify Publishing Group, especially production editor Myles Schrag, graphic designer Liam Brophy, and copy editor Tom Gresham for putting it all together in such an engaging, brain-friendly way.

MY SOCIAL SUPPORT NETWORK: I never felt alone while writing this book even though many days I was locked in my office researching and writing. I especially want to thank my amazing husband, David, and my two wonderful daughters, Alyssa and Ashley, who were my rock, my cheerleaders, and my sounding board. In addition, I'm so grateful to my sister Julie Watson, my sister-in-law Amy Smolensky, and my aunt, Margie Cooper, who were there for me day or night to help me stay Brain On! when I was stuck or discouraged. And finally, to my many friends and industry experts who continued to check in on me and root me on during this past year, especially Michelle Spehr, Ellen Rogin, Jen Arnold, Mim Senft, Carol Wagner, Michelle Rickard, Sarah Berkley, and Doreen Davis.

MY BRAIN ON! WORK HEROES AND (S)HEROES: A big thank you to all my wonderful NFP colleagues and leaders who I'm honored to call my work family. Words can't adequately express my heartfelt thanks to my manager, Kim Bell, who didn't hesitate to say yes when I approached her with my book idea and who has always supported and championed my passion projects and dreams. And to Rose Gregory, Rick Westfall, Jacob Boston, Tom Berno, and the entire NFP marketing, writing, and social team for supporting me and guiding me through this entire project. I also want to thank my other incredible managers, Mike Schneider and Shawn Ellis, who continue to ensure I'm given opportunities to grow and contribute in ways that align with my passion, strengths, and vision. To NFP's entire executive leadership team and HR team, including Doug Hammond, Mike Goldman, Eric Boester, Ed O'Malley, Mike James, Suzanne Spradley, Ginette Quesada-Kunkel, Mary

Steed, Pamela Wheeler, and Chris LaMour, who continue to model and ensure NFP is a Brain On! Regenerative organization. Finally, I'm so lucky to work with the best team of well-being experts and humans I know. They support me every day and help our clients create Brain On!, Energizer cultures across the globe.

MY INCREDIBLE TEACHERS: Beyond the amazing thought-leaders I've cited throughout my book, I want to specifically thank those industry leaders I've had the opportunity to learn from and interact with throughout the years. They have greatly influenced my personal life and work and include: Daniel H. Pink, Dr. David Rock, Dr. Evian Gordon, MD, PhD, Dr. Amishi Jha, Kelly McGonigal, PhD, Jeremy Hunter PhD, C. Otto Scharmer, Chip Conley, Michelle Maldonado, Lisa Lahey EdD (HGSE), Scott Shute, Daniel Goleman PhD, Tom Rath, Chade-Meng Tan, Dr. Martin E.P. Seligman, Dr. Darren Weissman, Jim Dethmer, Marc Brackett PhD, Sharon Salzberg, Rick Hanson PhD, Daniel G. Amen, MD, Ron Friedman PhD, Byron Katie, Tim Ryan, Arianna Huffington, Bruce H. Lipton PhD, Raj Sisodia PhD, Jon Kabat-Zinn PhD, Dr. Daniel J. Siegel, Janice Marturano, Dr. Joel Bennett, Mari Ryan, Brian Luke Seaward PhD, Dr. Debra Lafler, Laura Putnam, Ron Goetzel, Claude Silver, Eric Langshur, Judd Allen PhD, Dr. Rosie Ward, and Jennifer Pitts PhD.

MY PERSONAL DREAM TEAM: Every day, I give thanks for my amazing dream team of experts, healers, teachers, thought leaders, and organizations who really have helped me over the years get mentally stronger each and every day. This list includes: Dr. Timothy

Voll, Laura Rategan, Stephanie Meis, Cindy Perloff, Maya Marcia Wieder, Debra Poneman, Molly Zaremba, Gabby Bernstein, Dr. Amanda Holly, Dr. Donald Zimmerman, Dr. Debra Ehrlich, Nancy Marder and Infinity Foundation, The Bloomberg Institute, Dr. Steven Best, Mo Edjlali and Mindful Leader, the Inner MBA program, Wisdom 2.0, NeuroLeadership Institute, National Wellness Institute, WELCOA, *American Journal of Health Promotion,* and the entire team at Resolute Public Affairs.

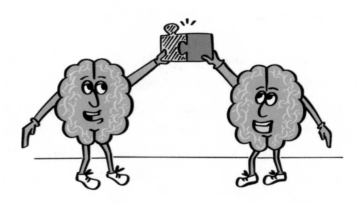

RESOURCES

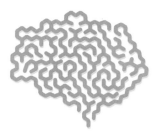

May you experience the many benefits that come when you exercise your brain for the purpose of a better workday and a better world.

It has been an honor serving as your mental fitness trainer. I hope you will continue to stay connected and use the resources in this book as well as on my website. There you'll find additional information for both you and your organization to stay mentally strong.

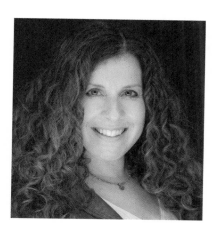

DEB SMOLENSKY is a highly sought-after author, speaker, and award-winning thought leader in the area of human performance and health at work. She serves as a Global Well-Being and Engagement Practice Leader and also as an advisor for the insurtech, fintech, and digital health start-up communities. Over the past twenty-five years, Deb has received numerous certifications and designations in organizational health and productivity. She consults with a variety of clients, including numerous Fortune 500 companies, to develop strategies, programs, and practices that empower employees and executives to lead healthy, productive lives at work through innovative, meaningful, and engaging solutions.

debsmolensky.com

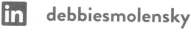 debbiesmolensky